Dr Penny Stanway practised for several years as a GP and as a child-health doctor before becoming increasingly fascinated by researching and writing about a healthy diet and other natural approaches to health and well-being. She is an accomplished cook who loves eating and very much enjoys being creative in the kitchen and sharing food with others. Penny has written more than 20 books on health, food and the connections between the two. She lives with her husband in a houseboat on the Thames and often visits the south west of Ireland. Her leisure pursuits include painting, swimming and being with her family and friends.

By the same author:

The Miracle of Lemons
The Miracle of Cider Vinegar
The Miracle of Bicarbonate of Soda
  (*US – The Miracle of Baking Soda*)
The Miracle of Olive Oil
The Miracle of Garlic
The Miracle of Honey
The Miracle of Spices
The Natural Guide to Women's Health
Healing Foods for Common Ailments
Good Food for Kids
Free Your Inner Artist
Breast is Best (new US edition called *The Breastfeeding Bible*)

As co-author:

Christmas – A Cook's Tour
The Lunchbox Book

THE MIRACLE OF
TEA

PRACTICAL TIPS FOR
HEALTH & HOME

DR PENNY STANWAY

WATKINS PUBLISHING
LONDON

This edition first published in the UK and USA 2013 by
Watkins Publishing Limited, Sixth Floor,
75 Wells Street, London W1T 3QH

A member of Osprey Group

Osprey Publishing Inc.
43-01 21st Street
Suite 220B, Long Island City
New York 11101

1 3 5 7 9 10 8 6 4 2

Designed and typeset by Jerry Goldie Graphic Design

Printed and bound in China

A CIP record for this book is available from the British Library

ISBN: 978-1-78028-574-0

www.watkinspublishing.co.uk

Contents

To all the friends and family,
neighbours and strangers,
with whom I've enjoyed so very many
cups of tea.

Acknowledgements

With thanks and love to my husband, Andrew, for his enthusiasm for tasting teas, and for his common sense and expertise during our many discussions as I researched and wrote this book.

Introduction

Tea is a daily delight to billions of people around the world. Its bushes and trees originated in China 60–70 million years ago. At some time, people discovered that chewing and swallowing the fresh leaves of wild tea trees tasted good and boosted their energy. Back in the mists of time, someone thought to pour hot water over these leaves and drink the resulting brew. Tea-drinking was first documented some 2,500 years ago, and by about 2,000 years ago, the drink was held in such high esteem that it was reserved only for emperors and other VIPs.

Around 1,500 or so years ago, green tea was being drunk by ordinary people and had become a locally traded commodity. The practice of oxidising green tea to make black tea, or fermenting it to make *puerh* tea, began during the Ming Dynasty (1368–1644). This allowed tea to stay wholesome when transported over long distances – for example, the 930 miles (1,500km) to Tibet along what became known as the 'Tea Road'.

Portuguese traders took green tea to Europe in the 1580s; the Dutch took tea to New Amsterdam (later New York) around 1650, and to England in 1669. In the 1860s, an undercover agent of England's East India Company leaked to India the secret of how black tea was made.

Black tea soon became the favourite in Europe and India, but green tea has remained the first choice in eastern Asia. This explains why it's the second most popular drink after water in the world.

All the while, peoples in different parts of the world were also using, enjoying and learning about herb teas – 'teas' made from other plants.

This book discusses the flavours, contents and uses not only of ordinary tea but also of a selection of herb teas, including everyday ones such as roasted barley, chamomile, peppermint and rooibos teas.

Not only can tea and certain herb teas be enjoyed as drinks, but they can also be useful beauty aids, delicious in recipes and good for our health.

CHAPTER ONE

Tea

The habit of tea-drinking is deeply embedded in many cultures, whether as a quick and restorative pick-me-up, for leisurely enjoyment, or during a calming, contemplative Japanese tea ceremony.

A staggering two billion cups of tea are drunk each day around the world, but the amounts vary country by country:

The brew we call tea originates from the downy leaf buds and thin leathery leaves of *Camellia sinensis*. Tea bushes and trees are cultivated mainly in tea plantations, known as gardens, in China, India and Japan, but also in certain other countries, including Kenya, Malawi, Nepal, Sri Lanka, Taiwan and Vietnam.

The genetic characteristics and age of these evergreens affect the constituents and the flavours of the brews made from them. Their geographical location or *terroir* (influenced by soil, altitude, latitude, climate and weather) is important, too. For just as the terroir of grapevines and olive trees affects the quality and nature of the wines and olive oils produced from them, so too does that of tea bushes and trees affect those of tea. Tea bushes and shrubs need an acidic, well-drained soil rich in minerals and humus and plenty of rain. Other variables are harvesting, processing and storage.

Highly prized premium or imperial teas mostly originate from the

TABLE 1: TEA-DRINKING PER CAPITA PER YEAR IN A SELECTION FROM 155 COUNTRIES*

Country	Dry tea: kg (oz)	Ranking
United Arab Emirates	6.24 (220)	1st
Morocco	4.34 (153)	2nd
Ireland	3.22 (114)	3rd
UK	1.89 (67)	7th
Russia	1.21 (43)	15th
China	0.82 (29)	33rd
New Zealand	0.65 (23)	45th
India	0.52 (18)	53rd
Australia; South Africa	0.52 (18)	joint 55th
Canada	0.41 (14)	62nd
US	0.33 (12)	69th
Germany	0.23 (8.1)	83rd
France	0.21 (7.4)	88th
Brazil	0.018kg (0.63)	142nd

* (United Nations' Food and Agriculture Organisation)

youngest buds, shoots and leaves, hand-plucked in early spring from the first flush of new growth of bushes at high altitudes. Such teas are particularly aromatic and have good, rich flavours.

Other names

Camellia sinensis, also called *Thea sinensis,* belongs to the botanical family of plants called tea. It has more than 3,000 subvarieties and cultivars, but just two main varieties: *Camellia sinensis* var. *sinensis,* the small-leaf 'China bush' that is resistant to cold temperatures, and

Camellia sinensis var. *assam*, the large-leaf 'Assam bush' that may become a tree, and needs plenty of warmth.

The word tea comes from *tay* in the *Min Nan* language of parts of China and Taiwan. Variations include *thé* in French and *té* in Spanish. *Cha* is Mandarin for tea in China and a nickname for tea in English-speaking countries. Japan and Portugal also use the word *cha*, while versions of it include *chai* in India and Russia.

Tea and *cha* derive from *tu* and *jia* in different languages of ancient China, both of which come from the even older *d'a*.

Harvesting

Plucking is done with shears, a motor-powered cutter or an industrial harvester. Hand-plucking is least damaging and therefore the least likely to trigger oxidation (*see* page 5), making it particularly useful for producing green teas. It takes 10lb (4.5kg) of fresh tea leaves to produce 2lb (0.9kg) of dried tea.

Plucking is done in spring and summer and, latitude and climate permitting, autumn or even winter. Certain teas are plucked several times a year (at most every three weeks), others only once, in spring. In China, the first spring growth, before the Qingming Festival on April 6, produces sought-after pre-Qingming teas. These are particularly sweet and aromatic and have relatively high levels of caffeine and polyphenol pigments called catechins. Their Japanese counterparts are *Shincha* green teas.

Plucking may be of:
- **Buds-only**: these are leaf buds, not flower buds. Their covering of downy hairs may make them look silvery or golden. Buds are

often called 'tips', and bud-rich – or 'tippy' – tea is highly prized.

- **Budsets**: a bud and one leaf, or a bud and two leaves. Budset-only tea is sometimes called pekoe tea (from the Chinese *Pak-ho*, meaning a baby's downy head). Plucking of a bud and one leaf is an 'imperial' or 'superfine' pluck; that of a bud and two leaves, a 'fine' pluck. The more buds in a tea, the sweeter and more aromatic its brew.

- **Longer shoots**: plucking of a bud and three leaves is a 'medium' pluck; that of a shoot with up to 5–6 leaves, a 'coarse' one. The lower the leaves on a shoot, the more mature they are, and the more different from younger leaves are the flavours of the brews made from them.

Types of tea

Freshly plucked tea leaves are processed in five main ways to produce the five main types of tea – black, green, oolong, white and *puerh*. Each type could be made from any tea bush or tree, but the China bush is favoured for green and white teas; the Assam for black.

Of all the tea produced around the world, 78 per cent is black, 20 per cent green and most of the remainder oolong. Only China produces all five types, although three-quarters of its total production is green. Almost all India's teas are black, and almost all Japanese ones green.

Tea processing

Each type of tea is produced with a particular number and combination of processes. The main ones are:

Withering – softens leaves. This helps them remain whole, retain their aromatic constituents and, when rolled, hold their shape. It also boosts sweetness by converting some of their content of complex sugars into simple ones and increases the range of aromatic compounds.

Rolling, tossing or tumbling – bruises leaves and twists or curls them, releasing and activating oxidation enzymes. A long, thin, well-rolled leaf is said to be 'wiry'.

Sifting – whole leaves are separated from broken ones and sifted into different sizes.

Machine-cutting – broken or lower-quality leaves are chopped into even-sized fragments. The regularity of size of such fragments later allows their constituents to infuse into water at the same rates, enabling predictable steeping times and flavours for their brews.

Oxidation – this enzyme-enabled chemical process is the main factor that differentiates teas. It is sometimes mistakenly called fermentation. Oxidation of chlorophyll removes the leaves' green colour. Oxidation of polyphenols called catechins into pigments called theaflavins and thearubigins gives the leaves red and brown colours and makes them less astringent. Theaflavins are more astringent than thearubigins.

Different degrees of oxidation produce different types of tea:
- Black and *shou puerh* teas are completely oxidised, therefore poorest in catechins and richest in theaflavins and thearubigins.
- Oolong and white teas are partially oxidised, so have middling amounts of catechins and thearubigins. White teas have middling amounts of theaflavins; oolongs none, though they do contain thearubigins from other sources.
- Green and *shen puerh* teas are not oxidised, so are richest in catechins and poorest in theaflavins and thearubigins.

Firing or steaming – heating to dry leaves; halts oxidation if necessary;

prevents fermentation by killing bacteria and fungi. The higher temperatures used for certain types of tea affect their flavour by creating new aromatic compounds, increasing carboxylic acids, caramelising sugars and producing complex and nutty or otherwise attractively flavoured constituents called Maillard-reaction compounds.

Fermentation – to reduce the leaves' bitterness and encourage sweetness and mellowness.

Ageing – to develop their flavour further.

Black teas

Mainly produced in India, Sri Lanka and Kenya, black teas constitute about 90 per cent of the tea drunk in Europe and the US, and are the most common teas drunk in India and the Middle East.

Their processing includes withering, rolling, sifting, complete oxidation, firing and, perhaps, ageing. Complete oxidation makes the leaves copper or bright gold in colour, and the particular degree of firing makes them black or dark brown.

Whole-leaf teas are sometimes graded as:

- Orange pekoe: longer, more mature leaves and no buds. The best, 'OP1', has more delicate leaves. Dutch merchants dubbed pekoe tea 'orange' in honour of the princes of Orange.
- Flowery orange pekoe: higher-quality tea, with shorter, younger leaves and some two-leaf budsets that give floral flavour notes.
- Golden flowery orange pekoe: even better tea, with some early-season budsets turned golden by oxidation.
- Tippy golden flowery orange pekoe: the finest tea, rich in budsets. The very finest tippy tea – 'special finest tippy golden flowery orange pekoe', or SFTGFOP 1 – has the highest (25 per cent) content of buds.

Broken-leaf teas are sometimes graded as broken orange pekoe, golden broken orange pekoe and tippy golden broken orange pekoe.

Black teas have the strongest body, flavour and astringence. They include:

Assam – from north eastern India, these make strong, dark brown brews that taste malty, biscuity and slightly bitter; they may be astringent or even slightly pungent. Often blended, they account for up to 75 per cent of India's tea production.

Ceylon – Sri Lankan teas that make a mid-brown brew with an intense, rich flavour. Some of these teas are described as 'pointy' because of their desirable brightness and acidity.

Darjeeling – Indian teas from the foothills of the Himalayas in West Bengal and made from a fine pluck (a bud and two leaves). Their brews are golden brown, with a delightfully aromatic scent and a delicately fresh flavour with some sweetness and, perhaps, notes of almonds and muscatel grapes. Darjeelings are known as the champagne of teas and account for only about 1 per cent of India's tea.

Yunnan Golden Buds (*Dian Hong*: 'buds of gold') – Chinese teas from Yunnan province, with buds and leaves, and fragrant notes of honey and pear.

Keemun (from the English for *Qimen*) – Chinese teas from Qimen county in Anhui province, with thin black leaves, little astringency and a rich, smooth, sweet, fruity flavour. *Keemun Mao Feng* teas are fine-plucked and have flavour notes of chocolate and earth.

Lapsang Souchong (*Zhengshan Souchong*: 'Middle-Mountain Small-Leaf Variety') – the world's oldest black teas, from China and, now, Taiwan. Their large leaves, the third and fourth on a shoot, are dried over burning pine, giving a smoky, slightly pungent flavour. 'Tarry' lapsangs are smoked over pinewood tar, so have tarry notes. The term 'China tea', familiar to many older people, generally means a smoky-flavoured black tea from China, such as this one.

Nilgiri – teas from the Nilgiri Hills in southern India. 'Frost teas', harvested in winter, are the finest, with a dark colour, an intensely aromatic fragrance, and a fresh, rich flavour with notes of fruit and spice and a lingering finish.

Green teas

These are mostly produced in China and Japan and account for most of the tea drunk there, but only 20 per cent or so of that in Europe and the US. They are also popular in North Africa and South America. Apart from the powdered varieties, they consist of whole leaves.

Their processing includes withering, firing, rolling, tossing or tumbling and sifting. In Japan, the leaves are steamed rather than fired to prevent oxidation. Rolled budsets, called 'swords' or 'needles', may float upright in a cup of tea. Rolled leaves are described as 'blades', 'strips' or 'twists'. Tumbling forms leaves into balls called 'pearls', 'pellets' or 'semi-balls', depending on their tightness and shape. The smallest and tightest are best as their shape helps prevent their essential oil, and therefore their flavour, from evaporating. Some teas are tied into balls.

Green teas are more delicately flavoured and, perhaps, more bitter than black teas. They include:

Curled Dragon Silver Tip (*Pan Long Yin Hao*) – Chinese teas made from early-spring leaves and characterised by great depth of flavour.

Dragon's Well (*Lung Ching*) – these pre-Qingming teas are considered

CHAPTER 2

Other teas

This chapter contains character 'snapshots' of 26 teas. Some make enjoyable everyday drinks. Some are good in recipes, or for personal care, or home care. All are valued medicines.

Most are straw, golden, light olive or light brown in colour, while hibiscus tea is pinkish-red and peppermint tea greenish-brown.

These teas are made from various parts of plants:
- All aerial parts – lemon balm, passionflower, rosemary and verbena teas
- Flowers – calendula, chamomile, elderflower, hibiscus, lavender, linden, red clover and rosehip teas
- Fruits – rosehips and *Vitex agnus castus* teas
- Leaves – chickweed, dandelion, nettle, peppermint, rooibos, rosemary and thyme teas
- Roots and/or rhizomes – black cohosh, dandelion, dong quai, echinacea, ginseng and valerian teas
- Seeds – barley and corn teas

The 'Notable contents' sections below highlight the bioactive constituents that most characterise each tea: for more information, see Chapter 3.

Barley and roasted barley teas

Made from the hulled (pearl barley) or unhulled (pot barley or barley groats) grains of *Hordeum distchon*, a plant in the grass family.

Other names – *Barley tea* is called barley water in the UK.

Roasted barley tea is popular in Korea (as *boricha*) and Japan (as *mugicha*).

Flavour – *Barley tea*: sweetish and slightly bitter.

Roasted barley tea: 'toasty' and a little like coffee but not as bitter.

Notable contents – *Barley tea*: alkaloids (such as gramine and hordenine); betaine; the mineral selenium; the phytoestrogen trigonelline.

Roasted barley tea: as above, plus complex flavour constituents ('Maillard-reaction compounds') created by roasting.

Used for – *Barley tea*: everyday drink; medicine.

Roasted barley tea: everyday drink.

Black cohosh tea

Made from the rhizomes and rootlets of *Cimicifuga racemosa*, a perennial plant in the buttercup family.

Other names – black snakeroot; bugbean; rattleroot; squaw root (confusingly, also a name for blue cohosh).

Flavour – acrid and bitter.

Notable contents – acids (such as ferulic); flavonoids; glycosides (for example, actein, cimicifugoside, racemoside and ranunculin); phytoestrogens (including cimicifugin and formononetin); resin; salicylates.

Used for – medicine.

Calendula tea

Made from the flowers of *Calendula officinalis*, a plant in the daisy family.

Other names – bulls eyes; gold bloom; marigold; marybud; pot marigold.

Flavour – floral and sweetish, with hints of bitterness and pungency.

Notable contents – acids (including chlorogenic acid); aromatics (such as cadinene and muurolol); carotenoids (including lycopene, neoxanthine, violaxanthine and zeaxanthin); complex sugars (in mucilage); flavonoids (for example, kaempferol, quercetin and rutin); glycosides; resin; sterols (including taraxasterol); lupeol (a terpene).

Used for – beauty aid; medicine.

Chamomile tea

Made from the flowers of *Matricaria chamomilla*; *Matricaria recutita*, an annual plant in the daisy family.

Other names – German chamomile; *Matricaria recutita*, wild chamomile.

Flavour – pleasantly aromatic and slightly bittersweet, with an apple note.

Notable contents – aromatics (such as azulene, bisabolol and farnesene); choline; coumarins (including herniarin and umbelliferone); flavonoids (for example, apigenin, chrysin, luteolin, rutin and quercetin); glycosides; acids (for instance, valeric); salicylates; sesquiterpene lactones (*see 'Terpenes and terpenoids'*, page 51) called nobilin; tannins.

Used for – beauty aid; everyday drink; medicine.

Chickweed tea

Made from the aerial parts of *Stellaria media*, an annual wild plant in the carnation family.

Other names – adder's mouth; chick wittles; clucken wort; satinflower; skirt buttons; star weed; tongue grass; winter weed.

Flavour – slightly salty.

Notable contents – acids (including valeric); alkaloids; complex sugars (in mucilage); copper; coumarins; flavonoids (for example, apigenin, kaempferol and rutin); glycosides; quinones (emodin, parietin and questin); saponins; sterols (daucosterol and β-sitosterol); tannins; vitamin C.

Used for – beauty aid; medicine.

Cornsilk and roasted corn teas

Cornsilk tea is made from the pistils of the flowers of *Zea mays*, a plant in the grass family.

Roasted corn tea is made from corn's roasted kernels (seeds).

Other names – *Cornsilk tea*: also called maize-silk tea. *Roasted corn tea*: popular in Korea (as *oksusu cha*).

Flavour – *Cornsilk tea*: sweetish.

Roasted corn tea: slightly sweet.

Notable contents – *Cornsilk tea*: acids (such as ferulic); alkaloids (such as hordenine); allantoin; complex sugars; the phytoestrogen trigonelline; saponins; sterols (β-sitosterol and stigmasterol); tannins.

Roasted corn tea: as above, plus complex flavour constituents ('Maillard-reaction compounds') created by roasting.

Used for – *Cornsilk tea*: beauty aid; medicine.

Roasted corn tea: everyday drink; medicine.

Dandelion and roasted dandelion tea

Made from the roots, or roasted roots, of *Taraxacum officinale*, a plant in the daisy family.

Other names – *Dandelion tea*: blow-ball; *dent-de-lion* (lion's tooth); fairy clock; priest's crown; wet-a-bed.

Roasted dandelion tea is often called dandelion coffee.

Flavour – *Dandelion tea*: mild, pleasant, slightly bitter and slightly sweet.

Roasted dandelion tea: rather like weak coffee.

Notable contents – *Dandelion tea*: acids (caffeic, chlorogenic, gallic, hydroxyphenylacetic and quinic); carotenoids (such as lutein, neoxanthine, violaxanthine and zeaxanthin); choline; complex sugars (such as inulin and pectin, in mucilage); flavonoids (for example, cynaroside; luteolin and flavoxanthin); glycosides (such as taraxacin); gum and resin; minerals (especially copper and iron); phytoestrogens (such as the coumarin derivative coumestrol); saponins; sesquiterpene lactones, *see Terpenes and terpenoids*, page 51 (including amyrin, lactupicrin, taraxol and taraxerol); sterols (such as β-sitosterol, stigmasterol and taraxasterol); tannins.

Roasted dandelion tea: as above, plus complex flavour constituents ('Maillard-reaction compounds') created by roasting.

Used for – beauty aid; everyday drink; medicine.

Dong-quai tea
Made from the roots of *Angelica sinensis*, a plant in the parsley/carrot family.

Other names – angelica root; Chinese angelica; *dong kwai*; women's ginseng. Note that *Angelica archangelica* (*Angelina officinalis*, or European angelica) is a different species.

Flavour – aromatic, slightly sweet and slightly bitter.

Notable contents – acids (for instance, angelic, ferulic, myristic and succinic); aromatics (such as carene, carvacrol, limonene, linalool, paracymene, phellandrene, α-pinene, sabinene and safrole); complex sugars; coumarins (for example, angelicone, angelol, psoralens and scopoletin); phthalides (including butylidenephthalide and ligustilide); polyacetylenes; sterols (including β-sitosterol); tannins.

Used for – beauty aid; medicine.

Echinacea tea

Made from the roots and rhizomes of *Echinacea angustifolia* and other echinacea species, perennial plants in the echinacea family.

Other names – black samson; coneflower; Kansas snakeroot; purple coneflower; rudbeckia.

Flavour – aromatic, earthy and sweetish, then slightly bitter. Also, pungent (thanks to echinacin), causing temporary numbness and tingling of the tongue.

Notable contents – acids (including caffeic, caftaric, chlorogenic and cichoric); alkylamides; aromatics (such as humulene and vanillin); complex sugars (such as echinacin and inulin); flavonoids; glycosides (for example, echinacoside); polyacetylenes; resin; tannins.

Used for – beauty aid; medicine.

Elderflower tea

Made from the flowers of *Sambucus nigra*, a shrubby tree in the honeysuckle family.

Other names – black elder; bore tree; elder; hollunder; pipe tree; *sureau*.

Flavour – floral, sweetish and mildly astringent. Tea made from flowers that have been fully open for some time may be slightly bitter.

Notable contents – acids (such as caffeic, chlorogenic, coumaric, ursolic and valeric); complex sugars (such as pectin, in mucilage); flavonoids (for example, kaempferol, rutin and quercetin); phytoestrogens; polyphenols; sterols (including campesterol, β-sitosterol and stigmasterol); tannins.

Used for – beauty aid; everyday drink; medicine; recipes.

Ginseng tea

Made from the roots of *Panax ginseng*, a perennial plant in the ivy family.

Other names – Asiatic, Chinese, Korean, oriental or true ginseng. Interestingly, *panax* means 'panacea'. Siberian ginseng (*Eleutherococcus senticosus*) is a different herb.

Flavour – pleasant; slightly sweet at first, then bitter.

Notable contents – acids; aromatics (such as β-elemene); choline; complex sugars; glycosides; polyacetylenes; saponins (ginsenosides).

Used for – medicine.

Hibiscus tea

Made from the sepals of the flowers of *Hibiscus sabdariffa*, a shrub in the mallow family.

Other names – *bissap* or *bissop* (in West Africa, it's the national drink in Senegal); dah (in Mali); *flor de Jamaica* (in Latin America); *karkadé* (in Jordan, Egypt and Sudan); rosemallow; rosella (in Australia); roselle (for example, in the Sahel); sorrel (in the West Indies).

Flavour – sour and slightly bitter, fruity and sweet (rather like cranberry).

Notable contents – acids (including citric, hibiscic, malic, protocatechuic and tartaric); an alkaloid; complex sugars; flavonoids (for example, cyanidin and delphinidin); phaseolamin; resin.

Used for – beauty aid; everyday drink; medicine; recipes.

Lavender tea
Made from the flowers of *Lavendula angustifolia*, a shrub in the mint family.

Flavour – strongly aromatic, slightly sweet.

Notable contents – acids (including caffeic and ursolic); aromatics (mainly linaloöl and linalyl acetate; also including β-caryophyllene, farnesene, ocimene, perillyl alcohol and terpinen-4-ol); coumarins (for example, coumarin, herniarin and umbelliferone); flavonoids (for example, luteolin); tannins.

Used for – beauty aid; ingredient in everyday herb tea blends; medicine; recipes.

Lemon-balm tea
Made from the aerial parts of *Melissa officinalis*, a herb in the mint family.

Other names – balm; bee balm; cure-all; honey plant; melissa; sweet balm.

Flavour – aromatic and slightly lemony.

Notable contents – acids (especially rosmarinic, also including caffeic, chlorogenic, pomolic, protocatechuic and ursolic); aromatics (mainly citral and citronellal; also including β-caryophyllene, citronellol, geraniol, linaloöl, nerol and ocimene); flavonoids (for example, apigenin, kaempferol, luteolin and quercetin; glycosides; resin; the mineral, selenium; tannins.

Used for – common ingredient of everyday herb tea blends; medicine; recipes.

Linden-blossom tea

Made from the flowers of trees in the tilia family.

Other names – till tree blossom.

Flavour – notes of honey and lime; slightly pungent.

Notable contents – acids (including caffeic, chlorogenic and coumaric); aromatics (mainly farnesol); flavonoids (for example, asparadin, hesperidin, kaempferol, quercetin and rutin); complex sugars (in mucilage); glycosides (such as astragalin and tiliroside); gum; saponins; tannins.

Used for – beauty aid; common ingredient in everyday herb tea blends; medicine.

Nettle tea

Made from the young tops and roots of *Urtica dioica*, a perennial wild plant in the nettle family.

Other names – stinging nettle.

Flavour – pleasant, and slightly grassy, salty and bitter.

Notable contents – acids (including formic, responsible for stinging by fresh leaves, but inactivated when making tea); amines (such as acetyl choline – *see 'choline and acetylcholine'*, page 42; histamine; and serotonin); betaine; complex sugars (in mucilage); coumarins (for example, scopoletin); flavonoids (for example, kaempferol, quercetin, rhamnetin and rutin); glycosides; minerals (for instance, calcium and iron); phytoestrogens; the pigment chlorophyll; a quinone (glucoquinone); sterols (for instance, β-sitosterol); tannins; vitamin D.

Used for – beauty aid; medicine.

Passionflower tea
Made from the aerial parts of *Passiflora incarnate*, a perennial climbing plant in the passionflower family.

Other names – maypop; granadilla.

Flavour – mild and slightly floral.

Notable contents – acids (including chlorogenic); alkaloids (of the 'harmala' group: harmaline, harman, harmine and harmol); coumarins (including scopoletin and umbelliferone); flavonoids (for example, apigenin, chrysin, kaempferol, luteolin, orientin, quercetin, rutin, saponarin and vitexin); glycosides (such as passiflorine); gums; and sterols (for example, stigmasterol).

Used for – beauty aid; ingredient in everyday herb tea blends; medicine.

Peppermint tea
Made from the aerial parts of *Mentha piperita*, a perennial plant in the mint family. *Mentha spicata* (common mint, garden mint, spearmint) contains less menthol, but is a good substitute.

Flavour – minty, slightly sweet and pungent.

Notable contents – acids (including caffeic, chlorogenic, rosmarinic and ursolic); aromatics (such as menthol, menthone and menthyl acetate); carotenoids (including neoxanthine, violaxanthine and zeaxanthin); choline; flavonoids (for example, luteolin, menthoside and rutin); pigments (such as chlorophyll); resin; salicylates; tannins.

Used for – beauty aid; everyday drink; medicine.

Red-clover tea

Made from the flowers of *Trifolium pretense*, a creeping biennial or perennial wild plant in the pea family.

Other names – clover rose; purple clover; sugar bosses; trefoil.

Flavour – slightly sweet, salty and minty.

Notable contents – aromatics (such as furfural); coumarins (including coumestrol and medicagol); flavonoids (for example, pectolinarin, trifoliin and red clover's phytoestrogens); glycosides; pectin; phytoestrogens (such as biochanin, daidzein, formononetin, genistein, pratensein and trifoside); sterols (for instance, β-sitosterol); polyphenols (clovamides).

Used for – beauty aid; medicine.

Rooibos tea

Made from the leaves and stems of *Aspalathus linearis*, a shrubby plant in the pea family.

Other names – Massai tea; redbush tea.

Green rooibos tea is made from newly picked, quickly dried leaves.

Red rooibos tea is made from newly picked leaves allowed to oxidise.

Flavour – pleasant, sweet, sour, bitter and tea-like.

Red rooibos tea is sweeter than green rooibos tea.

Notable contents – acids (including alpha-hydroxy, caffeic, coumaric, ferulic, hydroxybenzoic, protocatechuic and vanillic); an alkaloid (cyclopine); aromatics (such as damascenone, geranylacetone, guaiacol and phenylethanol); flavonoids (for example, aspalathin, chrysoeriol, luteolin, nothofagin, orientin, quercetin and rutin); the mineral magnesium; phytoestrogens; tannins.

Green rooibos tea has twice the antioxidant activity of red rooibos tea, thanks to its higher levels of the flavonoids aspalathin and nothofagin.

Used for – beauty aid; everyday drink; medicine; recipes.

Rosehip tea

Made from the fruits ('hips') of *Rosa canina*, a shrub in the rose family.

Other names – dogrose.

Flavour – slightly fruity, sour, sweet and bitter.

Notable contents – acids (for instance, ascorbic, ellagic and malic); aromatics (such as vanillin); carotenoids (for example, lycopene, neoxanthine violaxanthine and zeaxanthin); complex sugars (such as pectin) in mucilage; flavonoids (including anthocyanins, quercetin and rutin); tannins.

Used for – beauty aid; common ingredient in everyday herb tea blends; medicine.

Rosemary tea

Made from the aerial parts of *Rosmarinus officinalis*, a shrub in the mint family.

Other names – compass plant; romero.

Flavour – aromatic, pleasant and slightly bitter.

Notable contents – acids (including rosmarinic and ursolic); alkaloids (such as rosmaricine); aromatics (such as borneol, camphene, camphor, β-caryophyllene, eucalyptol, limonene, linaloöl, pinene, terpineol, thymol and verbenol); carnosol (a diterpene, *see* '*Terpenes*', page 51); flavonoids (for example, apigenin, diosmetin, diosmin and luteolin); a quinone (rosmariquinone); resin; and tannins.

Used for – beauty aid; medicine.

Thyme tea
Made from the leaves of *Thymus vulgaris*, a small shrub in the mint family.

Flavour – aromatic, pungent and slightly bitter.

Notable contents – acids (including caffeic labiatic and ursolic); aromatics (mainly camphor, camphene, carvacrol, terpine-4-ol and thymol); flavonoids (for example, apigenen, kaempferol, luteolin and a 'bitter' called serpyllin); phytoestrogens; saponins; tannins.

Used for – beauty aid; medicine.

Valerian tea
Made from the roots of *Valeriana officinalis*, a perennial plant in the valerian family.

Other names – capon's tail; heal-all; *phu*; setwall; spikenard; vandal root.

Flavour – slightly spicy and unpleasant.

Notable contents – alkaloids (including actinidine, chatinine, skythantine, valerianine and valerine); aromatics (such as bornyl acetate, camphene, myrtenyl acetate, myrtenyl isovalerate and pinene); choline; flavonoids (for example, a catechin called epigallocatechin gallate); glycosides (including, in dried valerian, certain iridoids called valepotriates and valerenic acid); phytoestrogens; and tannins.

Used for – beauty aid; medicine.

Verbena tea

Made from the aerial parts of *Verbena officinalis*, a perennial plant in the verbena family.

Other names – vervain; holy herb; Juno's tears; pigeon's grass; simpler's joy; traveller's joy; wild hyssop.

Flavour – bitter and slightly sweet.

Notable contents – acids (such as ursolic); aromatics (such as citral, geraniol, limonene and verbenone); an alkaloid; complex sugars (for example, stachyose) in mucilage; glycosides (including iridoids such as aucubin, bastatoside, verbenin and verbenalin); phytoestrogens; sterols (including dihydroxy-sitosterol and p-sitosterin); quinones; saponin; tannins.

Used for – beauty aid; common ingredient in everyday herb tea blends; medicine.

Vitez-Agnus-Castus tea

Made from the berries of this shrub or small tree in the mint family.

Other names – Abraham's balm; monk's pepper; chasteberry; wild lavender; tree of chastity.

Flavour – slightly aromatic and bitter.

Notable contents – alkaloids; aromatics (such as bornyl acetate, β-caryophyllene, eucalyptol, farnesene, pinene and sabinene); a 'bitter' called castine; flavonoids (for example, casticin, chrysosplenol, cynaroside, kaempferol, luteolin, orientin, rhamnetin and isovitexin); glycosides (such as casteine); iridoids, including agnoside and aucubin); possibly phytoestrogens (as *Vitex agnus castus* has some oestrogenic activity); rotundifuran (a diterpene, *see* '*Terpenes*', page 51); tannins.

Used for – medicine.

CHAPTER 3

What's in teas

Bioactive constituents contribute to the flavour of tea and herb teas and promote health and healing. Their types and amounts vary with a tea's variety and *terroir*, the plant part and its maturity, and the harvesting, processing and storage of the tea.

Below you'll find explanations of what the main groups of bioactive constituents do in the body, plus their sources. If you prefer to skip the science, you'll find practical ways of choosing and using teas to treat common ailments in Chapter 6.

Italicising of a constituent indicates it has its own entry.

Acids – sharpen flavour and have various actions: for example, caffeic is antibacterial, antifungal, anti-inflammatory, antiviral, antioxidant and pain relieving. Chlorogenic may aid weight loss by reducing carbohydrate absorption. Ellagic and ursolic are anticancer (ellagic, for example, may encourage apotosis – cell 'suicide' – of cancer cells). Ferulic is antioxidant and anti-inflammatory; reduces cholesterol and blood fats; discourages atherosclerosis, diabetes, cancer and Alzheimer's; may improve sperm-cell motility and viability; and can lessen period pain by making womb contractions less powerful. Gallic is antibacterial, anticancer, antifungal, antiviral and blood-sugar-lowering. Rosmarinic is antioxidant and anti-inflammatory; it can also lower blood sugar, help relieve hay fever and help widen narrowed airways. Valerenic increases the actions of the calming neurotransmitter gamma-amino-butyric acid.

Acids include:

Amino acids

Alpha-hydroxy acids: citric (in hibiscus and tea); malic (in hibiscus, rosehip and tea); and tartaric (in hibiscus). Also in rooibos.

Carboxylic acids: angelic and myristic (in dong quai); ascorbic (in rosehip); formic (in nettle); fumaric (in tea); hibiscic (in hibiscus and rosehip); hydroxybenzoic (in rooibos); salicylic (in black cohosh, chamomile and peppermint); succinic (in dong quai, lemon balm and tea); ursolic (in elderflower, lavender, lemon balm, peppermint, rosemary, thyme and verbena); valerenic (in valerian); valeric (in chamomile, chickweed and elderflower); and vanillic (in rooibos). Also in passionflower.

Phenolic acids (see also *polyphenols*): caffeic (in dandelion, echinacea, elderflower, lemon balm, linden, peppermint, rooibos and thyme); caftaric and cichoric (in echinacea); chlorogenic (in calendula, dandelion, echinacea, elderflower, lemon balm, linden, passionflower and peppermint); coumaric (in elderflower, linden and rooibos); ellagic (in rosehip); ferulic (in black cohosh, corn, dong quai and rooibos); gallic (in tea); hydroxyphenylacetic (in dandelion); labiatic (in thyme); protocatechuic (in hibiscus, lemon balm, rooibos and tea); quinic (in dandelion); and rosmarinic (in lemon balm). Also in passionflower.

Alkaloids – many taste bitter. They may be analgesic, antibacterial, anticancer, antispasmodic or stimulant.

For example, caffeine, theobromine and theophylline are stimulant (they counteract the natural body tranquillizer adenosine). They widen airways. Caffeine increases concentration (*see* page 57) and boosts the activity of adrenaline (*see* page 87) and acetylcholine and dopamine (*see* page 89). It's possible that it may discourage Parkinson's disease. It also discourages 'belly fat' (which is associated with type-2 diabetes and metabolic syndrome).

Theophylline widens airways and arteries and reduces cholesterol.

Harman, harmine and hordenine act as monoamine-oxidase inhibitors. MAO inhibitors aid in the metabolism of feel-good neurotransmitters serotonin and norephinephrine, producing a sense of well-being and helping to reduce anxiety.

Theobromine and theophylline are antispasmodic. Trigonelline (a *phytoestrogen*) is anticancer, antimigraine, blood-sugar-lowering, cholesterol-lowering and sedative, and helps prevent tooth-decay bacteria sticking to teeth.

Alkaloids include: actinidine, chatinine, valerianine and valerine (in valerian); caffeine, theobromine and theophylline (in tea); castine (in *Vitex agnus castus*); *choline*; cyclopine (in rooibos); gramine and hordenine (in barley); hordenine (in cornsilk and passionflower); harman and harmine (in passionflower); rosmaricine (in rosemary); trigonelline (in barley and corn).

Allantoin – in cornsillk has moisturising, exfoliative, soothing and wound-healing properties on the skin.

Amines – some, including *acetylcholine* and *serotonin*, act as neurotransmitters (*see* also page 42).

Amino acids – include theanine (mainly in black and oolong teas). Formed from proteins during oxidation, theanine can enter the brain and boost the action of the neurotransmitters dopamine, gamma-amino butyric acid and serotonin (*see* page 53), for example, boosting concentration and mental relaxation. It also discourages 'belly fat' (which is associated with type-2 diabetes and metabolic syndrome).

Antioxidants and anti-inflammatories – help prevent or treat many ailments and include *carotenes*; *coumarins*; *flavonoids*, *glycosides*, *tannins* and other *polyphenols*; *salicylates*, selenium (*see* 'Other constituents'); vitamin C (*see* 'Other constituents'); and certain *acids*.

Aromatics – volatile, scented essential-oil constituents. Most are terpenes; some are also *acids*, alcohols, aldehydes, esters, ketones or *phthalides*.

Aromatics may be airway-relaxing (eucalyptol); antiallergic (azulene); anti-anxiety (borneol and linaloöl); antibacterial (carvacrol, carvone, citronellal, eucalyptol, geraniol, linaloöl and thymol); anticancer (limonene, perillyl alcohol and thymol); antifungal (limonene, linaloöl and thymol); anti-itching (menthol, when used topically); anti-inflammatory (azulene and β-caryophyllene); cholesterol-lowering (eucalyptol and perillyl alcohol); decongestant and 'cooling' (menthol, when inhaled); expectorant (bornyl acetate, eucalyptol, limonene, phellandrene and pinene); gallstone-dissolving (limonene); memory-boosting (pinene and pulegone); pain-relieving (β-caryophyllene and, used topically, menthol); sedative (citronellal, limonene and linaloöl); and wind/gas-relieving (carvone and menthol). Thymol increases the activity of the neurotransmitter gamma-aminobutyric acid. Traces of essential oil containing linalool (for example, in lavender tea) may have anticonvulsant properties, possibly thanks to linalool binding to the excitatory neurotransmitter glutamate (*see* page 43).

TABLE 2: AROMATICS IN VARIOUS TEAS

Aromatic	Scent and flavour	Type of tea
Azulene	'Green', herbal, slightly sweet	Chamomile
Benzaldehyde	Fruity	Tea
Bisabolol	Floral	Chamomile
Borneol	Camphor, pepper, pine, woody	Rosemary, tea
Bornyl acetate	Berry, camphor, menthol, woody	Valerian, *Vitex agnus castus*
Cadinene	Herbal, woody	Calendula
α-cadinol	Herbal, woody	Tea
Camphene	Camphor, menthol, musty	Rosemary, thyme, valerian
Camphor	Camphor	Rosemary, thyme
Carene	Citrus, sweet	Dong quai
β-caryophyllene	Earthy, spicy, sweet, woody	Dong quai, echinacea, lemon balm, rosemary, *Vitex agnus castus*
Carvacrol	Oregano	Dong quai, tea, thyme
Citral (neral or geranial)	Citrus, fruity, 'green'	Lemon balm, verbena,
Citronellal	Lemon	Lemon balm
Citronellol	Citrus, 'green', rose, sweet	Lemon balm
Damascenone	floral, fruity, 'green', spicy, tobacco, woody	Rooibos
β-elemene	Fresh, herbal	Ginseng
Eucalyptol (cineole)	Spicy, woody	Rosemary, tea, *Vitex agnus castus*
Eugenol	Carnation, spicy	Linden
Farnesene	Herbal, woody	Chamomile, lavender, *Vitex agnus castus*
Farnesol	Floral, 'green'	Linden

Aromatic	Scent and flavour	Type of tea
Geraniol	Citrus, rose, sweet	Lemon balm, tea, verbena
Geranylacetone	Floral, fruity, 'green'	Rooibos
Guaiacol	Carnation, leather, spice, vanilla, woody	Rooibos
Heptanal	Fruity, herbal, woody	Lavender
Hexanal	Apple, fresh, grassy, orange, woody	Lavender, tea
Humulene (α-caryophyllene)	Woody	Echinacea
Ligustilide	Aromatic, floral	Dong quai
Limonene	Oranges	Dong quai, rosemary, verbena
Linaloöl	Lavender, spicy, sweet	Dong quai, lavender, lemon balm, rosemary, tea
Menthol	Mint	Peppermint
Menthone	Mint	Peppermint
Menthyl acetate	Mint, rose	Peppermint
Methyl salicylate	Camphor, root beer, sweet, wintergreen	Tea
Muurolol	Herbal, honey, spicy	Calendula, tea
Myrtenyl acetate	Fruity, floral, violet	Valerian
Myrtenyl isovalerate	Pine	Valerian
Nerol	Rose, citrus	Lemon balm
Nerolidol	Citrus, floral, 'green', sweet, woody	Tea
Ocimene	Floral, herbal, sweet	Lavender, lemon balm
Paracymene (formerly cymol)	Citrus	Dong quai
Perillyl alcohol	Cardamom, cumin, floral 'green', woody, orange, sweet	Lavender
β-phellandrene	Mint	Dong quai

Aromatic	Scent and flavour	Type of tea
Phenyl acetaldehyde	Chocolate, floral, honey, spicy	Tea
Phenyl ethanol	Bready, floral, fruity, rose, sweet	Rooibos, tea
α-pinene	Camphor, pine, woody	Dong quai, rosemary, tea, *Vitex agnus castus*
β-pinene	Camphor, minty, pine, resinous, spicy, woody	Tea, *Vitex agnus castus*
Piperonal	Carnation, cherry, vanilla	Vanilla
Sabinene	Citrus, pine, woody	Dong quai, *Vitex agnus castus*
Safrole	Spicy	Dong quai
α-terpineol	Citrus, floral, lilac, pine, woody	Rosemary
Terpine-4-ol	Citrus, clove, earthy, woody	Lavender, thyme
Thymol	Thyme	Rosemary, tea, thyme
Vanillin	Vanilla	Echinacea, rosehip
Verbenol	Pine	Rosemary
Verbenone	Camphor, celery, menthol	Verbena

Bitter principles (*see* also page 16) – tasting these boosts appetite; improves digestion; discourages food allergy; aids detoxification in the liver; and can lower blood sugar (by regulating the hormones insulin and glucagon). They work only if tasted. Some are antibiotic, anti-inflammatory, cholesterol-lowering or white-cell boosting. Serpyllin, for example, boosts appetite, discourages food allergies (by improving the digestions of proteins); stimulates the flow of digestive juices; helps regulate blood sugar (by regulating the production of the pancreatic hormones insulin and glucagon); and encourages stomach emptying.

They include *alkaloids*; *coumarins*; certain *flavonoids*; *glycosides*; *iridoids*; *salicylates*; *saponins*; serpyllin (in thyme); certain *terpenes and terpenoids*; and *tannins*.

Carotenoids – *terpenes* that are *pigments*.

Catechins – *flavonoids* and *tannins* that adhere to proteins in bacteria and viruses, preventing them adhering to and harming cells. It's thought that catechins may discourage Alzheimer's disease, eye diseases (such as glaucoma), candida infection and osteoporosis. It may discourage 'belly fat' (which is associated with type-2 diabetes and metabolic syndrome). In particular, epigallocatechin gallate's anti-inflammatory effects inhibit excessive production of the COX-2 enzyme that encourages arthritis and cancer. It may also reduce weight by helping to convert calories into muscle rather than fat, by prolonging the metabolism-boosting action of noradrenaline (norepinephrine), and by reducing appetite. It reduces brain damage after a stroke.

Choline and acetylcholine – choline is an *alkaloid* and an essential nutrient. Our body uses it to make the neurotransmitter acetylcholine (*see* page 88). Choline is present in chamomile, ginseng, nettle, peppermint and valerian; and acetylcholine in nettle.

Complex sugars – include oligosaccharides and polysaccharides. Some are sweet; some act as soluble dietary fibre; and some (including inulin and pectin) are prebiotics. Prebiotics increase 'good' gut bacteria called probiotics (such as lactobacilli and bifidobacteria) and decrease potentially harmful ones. As prebiotics break down, they release short-chain fatty acids that aid digestion; boost immunity; discourage colon cancer, constipation, diarrhoea, inflammatory bowel disease and an irritable bowel; and help prevent high blood pressure, high cholesterol (by decreasing its absorption from the gut), high blood sugar, abnormal blood clots and fibromyalgia.

Complex sugars include echinacin (in echinacea); inulin (sweetish soluble dietary fibre: in dandelion); pectin (soluble dietary fibre: in dandelion, elderflower and rosehip); and stachyose (sweetish: in verbena). They are also present in barley, chamomile, corn, dong quai, ginseng, hibiscus and tea.

Coumarins – are often *bitter*; may be antibacterial, anticancer, anticoagulant, antifungal, anti-inflammatory, antioxidant and antispasmodic; and those called psoralens react with sunlight to help eczema and psoriasis.

Coumarins include angelicone, angelol and psoralens (in dong quai); coumarin (in lavender); coumestrol and medicagol (in red clover); herniarin and umbelliferone (in chamomile, lavender and passionflower); and scopoletin (in dong quai, nettle and passionflower).

Essential oil (volatile oil) – a non-greasy, scented, readily evaporating oil. Each plant's essential oil has up to 300 constituents, many of them bioactive, including *alkaloids*, aromatics, carotenoids, *glycosides*, *phthalides*, *phytoestrogens*, *plant sterols*, *polyphenols*, *saponins*, *terpenes and terpenoids*, and vitamin-E-like substances. Some are antibacterial, anticancer, antifungal, anti-inflammatory, antispasmodic, carminative, diuretic, expectorant or blood-vessel-dilating.

Flavonoids – antioxidants, most being *pigments* and others, including catechins and proanthocyanidins (types of *tannin* in tea).

Glycosides – salts of constituents such as *flavonoids*, *saponins* and terpenes; generally *bitter*, sometimes *sweet* and possibly antibacterial, anti-inflammatory, antispasmodic or diuretic.

They include actein, cimigoside, racemoside and ranunculin (in black cohosh); agnoside and casteine (in *Vitex agnus castus*); anthocyanins (anthocyanidin glycosides: *see 'Pigments'*); apiin (in chamomile);

echinacoside (in echinacea); certain *flavonoid pigments*; ginsenosides (steroidal *saponins* in ginseng); ginsenin, panaquilin and panaxin (in ginseng); certain *iridoids*; passiflorine (in passionflower); pectolinarin and trifoliin (in red clover); *saponins*; taraxacin (in dandelion); and vanillin (in echinacea). Glycosides are also in calendula, chamomile, chickweed, dandelion, elderflower, linden, passionflower and nettle.

Gums and resins – gums (as in dandelion, linden and passion-flower) contain *complex sugars*. Resins (in black cohosh, calendula, dandelion, peppermint, red clover and rosemary) are scented and contain diterpenes (*see* '*Terpenes*').

Certain gums and resins are antibacterial, anti-inflammatory, expectorant or wound-healing.

Iridoids – *terpene* derivatives ('monoterpene lactones'), including agnoside (in *Vitex agnus castus*); aucubin (in *Vitex agnus castus* and verbena); bastatoside, verbenin and verbenalin (in verbena); valepo-triates (in valerian); and valerenic acid (in valerian).

They are the most bitter of the *bitter principles* and may be antispasmodic and calming (valerenic acid – which calms by increasing the action of the calming neurotransmitter gamma-aminobutyric acid, *see* page 89); anticancer and sedative (valepotriates); diuretic (aucubin); or laxative (asperuloside and aucubin). Valerenic acid also boosts the activity of the neurotransmitter gamma-aminobutyric acid.

Mucilage – made of *complex sugars* called polysaccharides, uronic acid and water, this slippery 'demulcent' gel soothes and protects inflamed or wounded skin, and mucous membrane in the gut, lungs, throat and urinary passages. It is antibacterial; reduces appetite (by increasing the feeling of fullness); and may lower blood sugar and cholesterol.

Mucilage is in calendula, chickweed, dandelion, elderflower, linden, nettle, rosehip and verbena.

Phthalides – widen blood vessels and include butylidenephthalide and ligustilide in dong quai. They may also have other actions: for example, ligustilide (also an *aromatic*) has anticlotting and anti-inflammatory actions, and boosts acetylcholine (*see* page 42).

Phytoestrogens – help balance high or low levels of our own oestrogens by attaching to and thus activating our cells' oestrogen receptors:

- In a woman with high oestrogen, phytoestrogens attaching to oestrogen receptors prevent her oestrogens attaching. Because hers would have been more strongly oestrogenic, this decreases her body's overall oestrogenic activity. This can help if an oestrogen-dominant hormone imbalance is causing bloating, cyclical weight gain, endometriosis, fibroids, heavy or irregular periods, infertility, irritability, lumpy tender breasts, miscarriage, nausea, polycystic ovary syndrome, post-menopausal bleeding, vaginal discharge, or womb, ovary or breast cancer.
- In a woman with low oestrogen (for example, after the menopause), phytoestrogens attaching to oestrogen receptors increase her body's overall oestrogenic activity. This can be helpful if oestrogen deficiency is causing acne, depression, dry vagina, fatigue, greasy hair and skin, irregular periods, low sex drive, non-cyclical weight gain or abnormal hairiness.

Certain phytoestrogens are antibacterial, anticancer, antimigraine, blood-sugar-lowering or cholesterol-lowering.

Phytoestrogens include certain *alkaloids* (such as trigonelline: in barley and corn); *coumarin* derivatives (such as coumestans: in red clover); *flavonoids* (flavonols such as kaempferol and myricetin: in tea; and quercetin: *see* <u>Yellow</u> or <u>yellowish-green</u> '*Pigments*'; isoflavones such as biochanin, daidzein, formononetin, genistein, lignans, pratensein and trifoside: in red clover; and formononetin: also in black cohosh and tea); lignans (in tea); saponins (such as ginsenoside in ginseng; and others in calendula); and *sterols*. Also cimicifugin (a resin; also antiviral; in black cohosh).

Also in dandelion, nettle, rooibos, thyme, valerian, verbena and, almost certainly, though as yet unidentified, *Vitex agnus castus*.

Pigments – coloured teas include:

- <u>Carotenoids</u>: *antioxidants* such as β-carotene (yellow: in dandelion and tea); lutein (yellow: in dandelion and tea); lycopene (yellow-orange: in calendula and rosehip); and neoxanthine, violaxanthine and zeaxanthin (reddish: in calendula, dandelion, peppermint, rosehip and tea).
- <u>Chlorophyll</u>: a green pigment claimed to act against cancer and help the body deal with toxins. Plentiful in nettle and peppermint teas and in green tea.
- *Flavonoid pigments*: *polyphenols* and *antioxidants*; some are also *glycosides*, *phytoestrogens* or *tannins*. They include dihydrochalcones, flavanones, flavanols, flavones, anthocyanidins and flavonols.

They can be analgesic, antiallergic, antibacterial, anticancer, antioxidant, antispasmodic, antiviral, astringent, *bitter*, diuretic, immunity boosting and sedative. Some reduce arterial stiffness (so improving circulation and reducing blood pressure), blood-clotting, blood sugar, and cholesterol; boost brainpower; improve vitamin-C absorption; aid inter-cell communication ('cell-signalling'); strengthen small blood vessels; and, perhaps, slow ageing. Many are anti-inflammatory and, unlike non-steroidal anti-inflammatory drugs, largely free from adverse effects. Many help protect collagen, the main protein in cartilage and connective tissue. They also discourage advanced glycation end products (AGEs) – formed by sugar joining with protein or fat during baking, roasting, grilling or frying, and associated with Alzheimer's, atherosclerosis (artery disease), arthritis, asthma, and diabetes.

They may be:

- **Yellow**: apigenin (in chickweed, lemon balm, passionflower, rosemary and thyme); aspalathin, chrysoeriol and nothofagin (in rooibos); astragalin, hesperidin and tiliroside (in linden); casticin, chrysosplenol and isovitexin (in *Vitex agnus castus*); catechins and myricetin (in tea); chrysin (in chamomile and passionflower); chrysosplenol (in *Vitex agnus castus*); cynaroside (in dandelion root and *Vitex agnus castus*); disometin and diosmin (in rosemary); biochanin, daidzein, formononetin, genistin, irilone, pratensein and trifoside (in red clover); kaempferol (in calendula, chickweed, elderflower, lemon balm, linden, nettle, passionflower, rosemary, tea and *Vitex agnus castus*); luteolin (in chamomile, lavender, lemon balm, passionflower, peppermint, rooibos, rosemary, thyme and *Vitex agnus castus*); orientin (in passionflower, rooibos and *Vitex agnus castus*); saponarin and vitexin (in passionflower); serpyllin (in thyme).
- **Yellow** or **yellowish-green**: quercetin (in calendula, chamomile, elderflower, lemon balm, linden, nettle, passionflower, rooibos, rosehip, rosemary, tea and valerian); rhamnetin (in nettle and *Vitex agnus castus*); rutin (in calendula, chamomile, chickweed, elderflower, linden, nettle, passionflower, peppermint, rooibos, rosehip and tea).

- <u>Yellowish-brown</u>: certain *tannins*.
- <u>Orange-red</u>: theaflavins (*tannins* in tea).
- <u>Pink, red</u> or <u>purple</u> (depending on a tea's acidity): anthocyanins (*see* 'Glycosides': in hibiscus, rosehip and tea); and anthocyanidins (such as cyanidin: in hibiscus; and delphinidin: in hibisucs and tea).
- <u>Red-brown</u>: theorubigins (*tannins* in tea).
- <u>Brown</u>: certain *tannins*.

In particular:
- Anthocyanidins reduce pain, reduce inflammation and nerve damage; help protect collagen; and taste astringent.
- Anthocyanins (*glycosides* of anthocyanidins) act against premature ageing, cancer, diabetes, bacterial infection, inflammation nerve damage and pain; are monoamine-oxidase inhibitors and so may help anxiety and depression (*see* page 85); they can also act like blood-pressure-reducing drugs called angiotensin-converting enzyme (ACE) inhibitors.
- Apigenin is antibacterial, anti-inflammatory, blood-pressure-lowering and diuretic.
- Biochanin, daidzein, formononetin, genistein, irilone, pratensein and trifoside are *phytoestrogens*.
- Catechins may be antispasmodic or sleep-inducing and encourage weight loss.
- Chrysin reduces pain and inflammation and may aid calmness and sleep.
- Chrysosplenol has antiviral action.
- Diosmin, hesperidin and rutin strengthen blood-vessel walls.
- Hesperidin is also cholesterol-lowering and anti-inflammatory.
- Kaempferol is analgesic, antianxiety, antiallergic, antibacterial,

anticancer, antidepressant, anti-inflammatory and antioxidant.

- Quercetin is anticancer, antidepressant, anti-inflammatory, antioxidant, antiviral and cholesterol lowering.
- Rutin is also antibacterial, anti-inflammatory and antiviral, and inhibits the formation of AGEs (*see* page 47).

Other pigments: include parietin (an orange-yellow quinone – see '*Other constituents*': quinone: in chickweed); pheophorbide (brownish: in tea) and pheophytin (blackish: in tea).

Polyacetylenes – are antibacterial, antifungal, anti-inflammatory, anticoagulant and, perhaps, anticancer. They are in dong quai, echinacea and ginseng.

Polyphenols – are anti-bacterial and antioxidant. Also, for example, clovamides (in red clover) help protect nerves from damage. They include certain *alkaloids*; *coumarins*; certain *essential-oil* aromatic terpenes and terpenoids (such as thymol in thyme); *flavonoids*; phenolic *acids*; and *salicylates*.

Salicylates – bitter salts of salicylic *acid*, with aspirin-like pain-relieving, anti-inflammatory, anticoagulant, anticancer and fever-lowering actions. They are in black cohosh, chamomile and peppermint.

Saponins – bitter, foaming triterpene (*see* '*Terpenes and terpenoids*'), steroid or steroid-alkaloid *glycosides* which act as expectorants (*see* page 100). Saponins are demulcent, so can soothe or protect inflamed or wounded skin or mucous membrane. Other possible actions include being antibacterial, antifungal, anti-inflammatory, blood-pressure-lowering, cholesterol-lowering, diuretic and wound-healing. They also may reduce appetite and lessen fat digestion by the enzyme pancreatic lipase.

Saponins include ginsenosides (steroidal saponins that are also *glycosides* and that can help regulate the body's steroid-hormone activity: in ginseng); and certain *phytoestrogens*. Also in cornsilk, dandelion, linden, nettle, thyme and verbena.

Sterols – types of triterpene (*see 'Terpenes and terpenoids'*) that can have antibacterial, antifungal, anti-inflammatory and other effects. For example, β-sitosterol has anticancer actions and reduces cholesterol and male-pattern baldness. It may discourage benign prostatic hypertrophy (BPH), because it reduces the hormone dihydrotestosterone and seems to equal finasteride (a BPH medication) in slowing prostate-cell growth. It may also discourage obesity, as it resembles fat in structure, so competes with fat for absorption from the gut.

They include β-sitosterol (in chickweed, corn, dandelion, dong quai, elderflower, nettle and red clover); campesterol (in elderflower); daucosterol (in chickweed); dihydroxy-sitosterol and p-sitosterin (in verbena); certain *phytoestrogens*; stigmasterol (in cornsilk, dandelion, elderflower and passionflower); and taxasterol (in calendula and dandelion). Also in nettle.

Sweet constituents – include certain *aromatics* (azulene, carene, β-caryophyllene, citronellol, geraniol, linaloöl, methyl salicylate, muurolol, nerolidol, ocimene, perillyl alcohol, phenylacetaldehyde and phenyl ethanol), *glycosides* and *polysaccharides*, as well as traces of simple sugars such as glucose, fructose, maltose (in Assam teas), raffinose and rhamnose (in China teas).

These give very slight natural sweetness to chamomile, dong quai, echinacea, elderflower, lavender, lemon balm, peppermint, rooibos, rosemary, tea, thyme, verbena and *Vitex agnus castus*.

Tannins – certain bitter *antioxidants*, *flavonoids* and *pigments* that can have antibacterial, anticancer, antifungal, anti-inflammatory, antiviral, blood-pressure- and blood-fat-lowering effects. They are astringent (*see* page 86), can harden skin, and might help diarrhoea and heavy periods.

Tannins include catechins; flavonoid-pigment precursors called proanthocyanidins; and flavonoid pigments (*see* '*Pigments*') called theaflavins and thearubigins.

They are in chamomile, cornsilk, dandelion, dong quai, echinacea, elderflower, lavender, lemon balm, linden, nettle, peppermint, rosehip, rosemary, tea, thyme, valerian and verbena.

Terpenes and terpenoids – fatty substances that include:

- Monoterpenes and sesquiterpenes: volatile and scented (*see* *Aromatics*).
- Diterpenes: scented and, perhaps, analgesic, antibacterial, anticancer, antifungal, anti-inflammatory and expectorant. Prevalent in resins (*see* '*Gums and resins*'). Also, rotundifuran, which can increase the action of the neurotransmitter dopamine (*see* page 89; in *Vitex agnus castus*).
- Triterpenes: lupeol (in calendula), *saponins* and *sterols*. Lupeol is antibacterial, antidiabetic, anti-inflammatory, antioxidant and painkilling. It also boosts collagen production (so aiding skin and connective-tissue regeneration and helping osteoarthritis); has anticancer properties; reduces prostate enlargement; and can help prevent or treat oxalate kidney stones.
- Tetraterpenoids: carotenoids (*see* '*Pigments*').

Their derivatives include:

- *Iridoids*.
- *S*esquiterpene lactones: these may be antibacterial, antifungal, anti-inflammatory, anticancer and cholesterol- and blood-fat- and blood-sugar-lowering and pain-relieving, and can

trigger allergic reactions in susceptible people. They include amyrin, lactupicrin, taraxol and taraxerol (in dandelion root); carnosol (which has antibacterial, anticancer, antifungal, anti-inflammatory and blood-fat-lowering properties: in rosemary); and nobilin (in chamomile).

Volatile oil – see '*Essential oil*'.

Other constituents – include proteins, carbohydrates, fats, minerals, vitamins and fibre. Their amounts are usually too small to be medically or nutritionally important. But barley and lemon balm are good sources of selenium (which may, for example, help prevent male infertility and prostate cancer); chickweed: vitamin C; dandelion: iron and copper; nettle: iron (indeed, it is richer in iron than spinach); rooibos: magnesium (which may aid its potentially calming effect); tea: fluoride (tea being an important source for many people) and manganese; and green tea (and, to a lesser extent, oolong, white and *puerh*): vitamin C.

Others include:
- Alkylamides (in echinacea) can bind to cannabinoid receptors on cells, reducing inflammation, pain and blood pressure; and have antibacterial, anticancer and antiviral properties.
- Betaine (in barley and nettle) is suggested to discourage heart disease by reducing high levels of the amino acid homocysteine.
- Maillard-reaction compounds: complex flavour constituents formed from sugars and protein when herbal matter is roasted. They include alkylpyrazines (which are thought to suppress appetite: in roasted barley); plus others (in roasted corn, roasted dandelion root and tea).
- Phaseolamin, a protein-like constituent of hibiscus tea that can aid weight loss by inhibiting amylases (starch-digesting enzymes) in the digestive tract.

- Quinones: can have anticancer, antibacterial, antioxidant, diuretic or other effects and include emodin, the orange-yellow *pigment* parietin and questin (in chickweed); glucoquinone (in nettle); and rosmariquinone (in rosemary). Quinones are also present in verbena.
- Serotonin, a neurotransmitter (*see* page 88) produced from melatonin (a hormone made at night after exposure to bright daylight in the day): in nettle (though in amounts probably too small to have much effect in the body). Whereas the serotonin made by our body within the brain has an antidepressant effect, any serotonin absorbed from a tea is unable to pass from the blood into the brain.

CHAPTER FOUR

Choosing, making and blending tea

Any cup of tea is fine if all you want is a hot tea-flavoured drink to perk you up and give you a break. But there's much reward to be had from experimentation, for tea varies hugely in its flavour, mouth-feel and how it's produced, as well as how it's brewed. Also, you may prefer a strong tea in the morning, more delicate teas throughout the day and a low- or no-caffeine tea in the evening.

About 3.5 billion cups are drunk each day around the world – about 165 million in Britain, where tea is more than twice as popular as coffee.

Teabags are by far the most popular format for tea in the West. In the UK, for example, an astonishing 96 per cent of tea comes as teabags. The other formats are loose, instant, compressed, bottled, canned and decaffeinated teas and, for special occasions, tea 'flowers'.

Loose tea
This contains loose whole leaves and is richest in flavourful and health-promoting aromatics. It generally comes in cardboard packets,

but tins, aluminised packaging and vacuum packing lengthen shelf life.

Teabags

In 1907, a US trader and distributor called Thomas Sullivan distributed samples of tea in small silk bags. People quickly realised they could put these straight into a pot. When effectively modified teabags were launched commercially – in 1949 in the US and in 1953 in the UK – they became an instant success.

Teabags are popular because they are quick and easy to use. Many of us steep a teabag for a very short time – perhaps 30 seconds or less. This may indeed be enough to get the optimal flavour from the tiny fragments, or dust, in cheaper teabags, but better-quality contents need longer.

At one time, most teabags contained mainly, or solely, fannings and dust left over from loose-tea production. These make poorer tasting teas than larger, even-sized machine-cut fragments or whole leaves, because their very large area of exposed surfaces means a proportion of their aromatics has already escaped.

Soon, though, the increasing demand for teabags, and the move away from loose tea, meant there weren't enough fannings and dust to meet the world's desire for teabags. Along with increasing consumer demand for high-quality tea, this led processors to increase their use of machine-cut leaves.

The similarity in size of these pieces enables their constituents to escape at a regular rate, which produces better-flavoured tea than that from fannings and dust. And their small size allows their constituents to infuse quickly into water, which suits our busy lives. But their large cut-surface area makes them less flavourful and faster to stale than whole-leaf tea. All types of tea are available in teabags.

Most teabags can make two cups. One-cup bags are also available.

Teabag size and shape – the best bags give their contents space to expand and 'dance' in the water. This maximises the brew's flavour and concentration of bioactive constituents. Teabags can be round, square or pyramidal. Some have a string with a tag for easy removal from the cup or a drawstring to extract water after steeping.

Teabag material – chlorine-bleached paper can release unpleasant flavours from traces of chlorine compounds. So many teabags are now made of oxygen-bleached or unbleached paper. The packaging may say 'TCF' (totally chlorine-free) or 'PCF' (processed chlorine-free). If it doesn't, you could contact the manufacturer to find out more. Pyramidal teabags are made of a synthetic, non-biodegradable material.

Buying empty bags or making your own teabags – when compared with purchasing ready-filled teabags, this may be cheaper and enable you to have better-quality tea for the same outlay.

Empty cotton teabags of various sizes are available on the Internet. Fill each one only half-full as a dried teabag expands when wet.

Or you could make teabags from muslin or cheesecloth secured with a lightweight string bow. Fabric teabags are washable and reusable.

Bottled and canned teas
These contain tea that's ready to drink; also good when chilled.

Compressed tea
This includes most *puerh* teas and tea bricks. To make tea from a larger *puerh* shape or a tea brick, you cut off a piece.

Instant tea

This powdered or granulated tea is used like instant coffee. Certain instant teas are flavoured, perhaps with fruit, honey or spices. Some contain powdered milk. But their flavour and content of health-promoting aromatics are unlikely to match those of other teas.

The question of caffeine (*see* also page 79)

Caffeine comprises around 3 per cent of the weight of dried tea, with brews made from young leaves, small fragments or Chinese tea containing most.

Caffeine boosts the actions of certain of the body's neurotransmitters, including adrenaline (epinephrine) and dopamine. Within 10–15 minutes this increases alertness, concentration and the feeling of satisfaction. Tea's tannins begin combining with caffeine after two minutes of steeping, so compared with caffeine from coffee it's released in the body more slowly, and its effects last longer.

TABLE 3: CAFFEINE CONTENT (IN MG) OF DIFFERENT DRINKS PER 8FL OZ (240ML) CUP *

White tea	10–25
Green tea	15–35
Hot chocolate	48
Oolong tea	15–50
Cola	Up to 50
Black tea	14–61 (on average, 40)
Cappuccino and instant coffee	24–173
Filter, cafetière and percolated coffee	95–200
Caffeinated 'energy drinks'	20–1368

* A 35ml serving of espresso coffee contains about 50mg.

Tea has less caffeine than most other caffeine-containing drinks.

Note that certain over-the-counter painkillers contain 15–65 mg of caffeine and some prescription-only versions up to 100 mg.

Tea's vitamin C (not found in black tea) and theanine (mostly in black and oolong teas) counteract some of the possible adverse effects of caffeine.

If you are caffeine-sensitive, ignore advice to 'rinse out' caffeine by steeping a teabag or tea leaves for 45 seconds and pouring away the resulting brew before steeping properly. Tests show this removes extremely little.

A good solution is to drink decaffeinated tea or an everyday herb tea.

Decaffeinated tea – decaffeination of black, green and oolong teas removes nearly all the caffeine and is done industrially:

With ethyl acetate, in which case 70 per cent of the tea's polyphenol content is lost. Or with water and carbon dioxide, in which case only 5 per cent of its polyphenol content is lost.

The latter is better, since polyphenols add flavour and promote health. Contact the manufacturer if a tea's packaging doesn't mention the method and you would like to know.

Tea flowers

These are made by sewing dried green-tea leaves together with dried flowers such as globe amaranth, hibiscus, jasmine, Chinese lilies or marigold. Steeping enables the 'blossoming' of a fantastic flower. This 'blooming' tea is best enjoyed in a glass teapot.

Making tea

Warm the cup, mug or teapot first by filling it with very hot water and letting it stand for a while. Or, if using high-quality tea, do a rapid first steep and discard the resulting brew before re-steeping properly.

If using loose tea, *either* put this into a mug- or teapot-infuser, *or* strain the brew, *or* hold the tea leaves back with a *gaiwan* lid while pouring out the brew (*see* 'Accessories', page 74).

How much tea?

You need different volumes of different teas, because although the required weight of any one is about 2–3g, larger-leaf teas take up more space than smaller-leaf ones.

You may choose to add slightly more or less, depending on the type of tea and the strength you want.

For green pearl tea, simply use 8–10 pearls per cup.

When making a pot of tea, it's traditional to use 1 rounded teaspoonful of tea per person and one 'for the pot'.

TABLE 4: AMOUNT OF TEA PER 6FL OZ (177ML) CUP

Type of tea	Teaspoons
Black whole-leaf or large-fragment	2
Black smaller-fragment	1
Green Chinese large-leaf	3–6
Green Chinese medium-leaf Green Chinese medium-bud	2–3
Green Chinese small-leaf Green Chinese 'pearl' Green Chinese small-bud	1–2
Green Japanese	1–2

Adding water

Hot water opens tea leaf pores and allows bioactive constituents to emerge from them and both the leaves' cut surfaces. Water-soluble constituents dissolve in the water; oil-soluble ones form tiny suspended droplets.

The four crucial factors are good-quality water; water whose temperature is appropriate to the tea; adding just enough water for a first 'round' of drinks; and neither over-steeping nor under-steeping.

The ideal water is:

- Neither too hard (calcium- and magnesium-rich, which increases tea's astringency and bitterness, darkens the tea and reduce its aromatics), nor too soft (mineral-poor, which makes tea taste 'flat'). If your water is hard, consider filtering it; using a tea specially blended and marked as appropriate for hard water; or boiling the water for several minutes. Also, keep your kettle descaled (by treating it with white vinegar when necessary), so flakes of scale can't despoil your cup of tea.
- Either pH 7 (a neutral acidity/alkalinity balance – pH) or very slightly acidic (pH just below 7), for optimal flavour and brightness of colour. If necessary, use a bottled spring water whose pH is 7, and with a total-dissolved-solids level lower than 30 parts per million). Or add a small pinch of bicarbonate of soda (baking soda) to the brew.
- Neither chlorinated nor distilled.
- Freshly drawn.
- Boiled once only, as reboiled water makes flat-tasting tea.

Water temperature – the optimal temperature varies with the tea. Too high and the brew is dark, bitter (because more tannins are released), and lacks optimal flavour and health-promoting properties (because

TABLE 5: IDEAL WATER TEMPERATURE FOR DIFFERENT TEAS

Type of tea	What to do	°C	°F	Look for
Chinese spring-harvested green; Japanese green; White	Heat water until just boiling, then let it cool for 5 minutes	65–70	149–158	
Most green; *shen puerh*	Heat water until just boiling, then let it cool for 3 minutes	75–80	167–176	A column of steam steadily rising from the water
Oolong *	Heat water until just boiling, then let it cool for 2 minutes	80–85	176–185	Large bubbles slowly rising and gently surfacing (the Chinese describe this as 'Fish Eyes')
Black	Heat water until just boiling, then let it cool for 1 minute	99	210	Almost-boiling water, with tiny bubbles surfacing around its circumference (the Chinese describe this as 'String of Pearls')
shou puerh	Heat water to a rolling boil and use at once	100	212	A rolling boil (the Chinese describe this as 'Turbulent Waters')

* If steeping oolong tea many times (see page 63), use slightly hotter water each time.

more of its aromatic content evaporates). Too low and its flavour notes don't develop properly.

Black and *shou puerh* teas need relatively hotter water to extract the large complex molecules of their flavourful oxidised polyphenols.

Green, oolong, white and *shen puerh* teas need relatively cooler water to preserve their colour and antioxidant power.

When making green, oolong or *shen puerh* tea, the reason for boiling then cooling the water, rather than heating it only to the required temperature, is that boiling drives off the oxygen dissolved in the water. This can't then oxidise polyphenols and thus changes the tea's flavour, reduces its antioxidant power and turns green tea brown.

Stirring or shaking

After adding water to dried tea, stir the leaves or gently prod the teabag(s) with a spoon. If using a teapot, give it a good shake, holding the lid on firmly.

Steeping

This extracts flavour, colour and health-promoting constituents from dried tea. The longer a steep, the greater the brew's content of caffeine and bitter and/or astringent polyphenols.

Black tea tastes best if covered while steeping so it retains its heat. Green tea is better steeped uncovered so it cools faster and can brew more gently.

To make a stronger brew, use a bigger volume of dried tea rather than a longer steep, since over-steeping increases bitterness and gives an unpleasant 'stewed' flavour. To make a weaker brew, use a smaller volume of tea rather than a shorter steep, since although each produces the same result, the former saves money!

How many steepings? – Black tea is widely considered best steeped only once, although some people refill a teapot, and some reuse teabags.

Other teas can be steeped several times. Each time, water penetrates the leaves further, releasing different flavours. With high-quality tea, the first steep can be a quick rinse to warm the container, clean the tea and, perhaps, reduce bitterness, before being discarded. Subsequent

TABLE 6: STEEPING TIMES

Type of tea	Time in minutes
White	1.5–2
Green *	Most are best with 2–3
Oolong	1–5 **
Black medium or small-leaf	2–3.5
Black tea large-leaf	3.5–5 ***
puerh	Limitless

* Some green teas are better steeped for only 30 seconds, others for up to 7 minutes.

** Shorter for 'semi-ball' oolongs; longer for 'needle' ones. The time also varies according to whether steeping Western or Asian style (*see below*).

*** A brew's antioxidant concentration peaks at 5 minutes; it's then 30 per cent higher than after 3 minutes' steeping, and 30 per cent higher than after 1 minute's.

TABLE 7: NUMBER OF STEEPINGS

Type of tea	Number of steepings
White	3 or more
Green	3–6
Oolong *	4–8 or more
Black medium or small-leaf	1
Black large-leaf	1; or 2 if steeped only briefly the first time
puerh **	Up to 10

* Aged oolongs can be steeped the largest number of times as they hydrate most slowly.

** A *puerh*'s first steep is just a rinse, with the water discarded; the second should be 25 seconds; for each steep from the third to the ninth, add 5 seconds; the tenth should be 90 seconds.

infusions are then drunk: the third, fourth and fifth are generally considered best. Ball-shaped green teas unfurl slowly so continue to release flavour over comparatively more infusions.

'Semi-ball'-shaped oolongs can be steeped more times than strip-shaped ones as they hydrate more slowly. The first steep should last 10–60 seconds; the second, 15–65 seconds; the third and others 5–10 seconds more for each steep, and an extra 30 seconds each as the flavour begins to diminish.

Tips for black tea – If using a teapot, after pouring out the first round of tea, avoid over-steeping any remaining tea by removing the leaves (which necessitates having a removable filter), or straining the brew into another, warmed pot.

Adding milk

Most people in dairying countries add cold fresh cows' milk to a brew of black tea. In the UK, for example, 98 per cent of people add milk. In India, people sometimes boil dried black tea *with* milk. The practice of adding milk is said to have begun in order to prevent hot tea cracking delicate porcelain cups. Milk isn't usually added to other teas and never to green tea. There is no right or wrong about adding milk – indeed, many tea connoisseurs add it. However, the flavour of tea with milk comes through best if the tea is strong. Add milk to tea, rather than tea to milk. You can then add just enough to give your preferred colour and flavour.

The advantages are that milk:

- Could make tea taste better to you by masking its bitterness and reducing its astringency.
- Adds sweetness (from its lactose – milk sugar).
- Adds nourishment (from its protein, fat, carbohydrate, minerals

and vitamins). Four cups of tea with milk provide one-fifth of the average adult's daily calcium requirement. Interestingly, older women who drink this much have better bone density than those who drink no tea.

- Neutralises tannins in tea, which would otherwise combine with calcium and iron in the gut and make them less readily absorbed (*see* page 50).
- Binds with oxalates in tea, reducing their absorption from the gut. This is good for 'stone-formers' – people with a propensity for forming oxalate kidney stones.
- Lowers the brew's temperature, which could discourage oesophageal and gastric cancers linked with heat damage from frequent consumption of very hot drinks or food.

The disadvantages are that:

- Milk proteins reduce tea's polyphenol content – and therefore its colour, flavour and health benefits – by up to 18 per cent, depending on the type and amount of milk. Skimmed milk has more protein (therefore greater polyphenol-lowering power) than semi-skimmed, which, in turn, has more than whole milk.
- Any masking of bitterness by milk's sweetness negates many of the health benefits of bitterness, as bitterness must be tastable to have these effects.

Some people use dried, evaporated or condensed milk, others camel, goat, horse, sheep or yak milk; lactose-free milk; almond, oat, rice or soy 'milk'; or cream. In Bhutan, Mongolia, Nepal and Tibet it's traditional to add yak butter for energy and flavour. Some nomads are said to drink up to 40 cups a day.

Blending

Black tea is frequently blended, including about 90 per cent of that drunk in the UK. Blenders may mix up to 35 teas to make an attractive blend. Favoured blends vary by country and even by region. Many people in the North of England, for example, like particularly strong black tea.

You can blend teas yourself by mixing loose teas.

Popular commercial blends include:

English Breakfast Tea – containing Assam, Ceylon and Kenya teas.

Genmaicha – a nutty-flavoured blend of Japanese green tree and dry-fried ('roasted') rice tea.

Irish Breakfast Tea – usually containing Assam teas.

Russian Caravan – smoky-flavoured blends usually containing *Lapsang Souchong* and often Oolong and Keemun teas.

Flavouring

Teas flavoured during processing include:
- Earl Grey teas (see page 15).
- Green Chinese teas scented with flowers of jasmine (*see* page 15), kwai (Chinese bay, giving a peach flavour), lotus, lychee or osmanthus.
- Green or black Chinese tea with roses.
- Persian rose tea – black tea with rosebuds and petals, borage and cardamom.

You could flavour teas, for example, with alcohol (a spirit or liqueur, or wine: for example, in punch – *see* page 126); chocolate or cocoa;

lemon juice (popular in black tea in eastern Europe, Italy and eastern India); herbs (such as basil or sage: popular in black tea in the Middle East); mint (popular in green gunpowder tea in North Africa); orange zest; or salt (popular in northern Pakistan, and Tibet).

Well-known flavoured teas include:

Lemon masala tea – this black tea with dry-fried cumin, lemon juice and black salt is popular in eastern India. Lemon, like milk, helps prevent tea reducing mineral absorption from food.

Masala chai – *see* page 124.

Russian tea – this is strong sweetened black tea simmered for 30 minutes with, for example, lemon, orange and pineapple juices, and a few cloves.

Frothy tea

In West and North Africa, tea is often poured from a height. This aerates it, producing a frothy head and altered flavour. In southeastern Asia, a mixture of black tea and condensed milk is sometimes poured from a height from one cup to another several times to make 'pulled' tea (*teh tarik*).

Avoiding scum

Certain brews develop a thin surface layer of scum. This consists of calcium carbonate plus organic substances and seems more likely in tea made from teabags. To discourage it, use loose leaves and filtered water, or add lemon (as its acid dissipates calcium carbonate).

Herb tea

Herbs are available fresh or dried, loose or in teabags, from supermarkets, grocers, specialist, ethnic or natural food stores, or online. Harvest them yourself only if you can identify them reliably and source them from land not recently treated with pesticides or herbicides. (The safe time between treatment and harvest varies with the product used.)

When travelling, taking herb teabags with you is an easy way to make your favoured drink.

Making herb teas

Choose the herb (or herbs for a blend) according to its format and availability, and whether you want the tea to be relaxing or stimulating, have health-promoting and/or healing actions, or offer a particular flavour.

When making a blended herb tea containing soft and hard herbal matter, prepare the herbs separately, using the appropriate methods below, then mix the resulting teas.

If you make more tea than you need, refrigerate the excess and use within 24 hours. After that it should be discarded, as spore-forming microorganisms are not effectively destroyed by boiling water.

Herb teas are almost always drunk without milk, roasted dandelion-root 'coffee' being an exception.

Use heaped amounts in teaspoon and tablespoon measures.

Using berries, cornsilks, flowers, 'thin' leaves or rosehips – for most teas:

To make 1 cup:

Put 1 teabag or 1 teaspoon of dried herbs (slightly crushed with a mortar and pestle, if necessary, or powdered) or 2 teaspoons of fresh, lightly chopped herbs into a cup. Add just-boiled water, steep for 10–15 minutes, then strain if necessary.

But for:

Chickweed tea – make tea from fresh chickweed.

Using roots, rhizomes, rosehips or seeds – for most teas:

To make about 3 cups:

- Put 1 tablespoon of dried plant matter or 2 tablespoons chopped fresh into a pan; add 4 cups of water; simmer, covered, for 10–15 minutes; steep for 10 minutes; then strain.
- OR soak 1 tablespoon of chopped or ground dried plant matter in 3 cups of just-boiled water, covered, for 12 hours; then strain and use within 12 hours.

But for:

Rosehip tea: use 15 whole dried or fresh and halved hips, or 6 teaspoons of crushed dried ones, for 3 cups of tea.

Valerian tea: steep 1 teaspoon of finely powdered dried root in 1 cup of just-boiled water for 10–15 minutes; then strain. (Boiling the roots would make a tea that smells and tastes unpleasant.)

Using roasted grains or roots – 'roasted' means dry-fried or oven-baked. You can buy roasted barley, corn or dandelion as powders or teabags. Or you can process the grains or roots yourself.

To dry-fry, cook them in a dry pan, tossing them frequently, for about 10 minutes or until fragrant and beginning to darken. To oven-bake, cook them at 150°C (300°F, gas 2), turning them occasionally until fragrant and beginning to darken. To grind cooled roasted grains or roots, use a pestle and mortar, a coffee grinder or an electric blender.

Roasted barley tea: is often served chilled.

To make about 3 cups:

- Simmer 1 tablespoon of roasted grains in 4 cups of water for 15 minutes; remove from the heat; steep for 5 minutes; then strain.

Roasted corn tea: remove kernels from corncobs, reserve the 'bare' cobs and roast the kernels as above.

To make about 3 cups:

- Put 1 tablespoon of roasted kernels, the bare cob and 5 cups of water in a large pan; simmer for 50 minutes until the brew is pale yellow; remove the cobs; and strain. Serve the tea with a few kernels in each cup.

Roasted dandelion-root tea (dandelion 'coffee')

To make about 3 cups:

- Simmer 1 tablespoon of roasted chopped dried root in 4 cups of water for 10 minutes.

Blends and flavourings for herb tea

Commercially available blends come as teabags and dried mixes.

You can also blend leaves, grains and roots yourself. If certain herbs in your chosen blend require simmering and steeping, others just steeping, simmer those that require simmering; add the others; then steep them together.

Good combinations include:

- Roasted barley and roasted corn teas (corn's sweetness reduces barley's bitterness).
- Chamomile tea, and tea.
- Elderflower and either lemon balm or peppermint teas.
- Lemon balm tea, and either elderflower tea, or tea.
- Nettle tea, and tea.
- Peppermint and green teas.
- Rosehip and hibiscus teas (hibiscus boosts rosehip's slight pinkness and adds lemony notes to rosehip's tartness).

Other flavours to consider adding as a tea brews include dried apple, cocoa, lemon or orange zest, or spice. Tried and tested additions include, for:

Barley tea: ginger, lemon, mint or orange.

Chamomile tea: dried apple, or cinnamon, ginger, vanilla or peppermint.

Chickweed tea: lemon or orange.

Dandelion tea: cinnamon.

Ginseng tea: ginger and lemon, or liquorice.

Hibiscus tea: cinnamon, clove, ginger, lemon, mint or nutmeg.

Lemon balm tea: lime juice or mint.

Nettle tea: blackberry or peppermint.

Peppermint: cocoa.

Rooibos tea: cocoa or lemon.

Hot or cold?

'True' teas, certain flavoured teas and many herb teas are good hot or cold. Lemon tea is particularly good iced, as are roasted corn, hibiscus, peppermint and rooibos teas.

Sweetening tea or herb tea

Adding sugar is very popular – in the UK, for example, nearly one in three people do it. Some of us sweeten a tea because we like it or to disguise bitterness (*see* page 41). The most popular sweetening in the West is white table sugar.

Unrefined sugar is an alternative, as are agave nectar, apple juice, honey, jam (popular in Russia), maple syrup and stevia (a plant extract whose glycosides are up to 300 times as sweet as sugar, but raise blood sugar hardly at all). Cardamom, cinnamon, ginger, liquorice, nutmeg, and vanilla can also contribute slight sweetness.

Tea and certain herb teas are naturally slightly sweet, with corn being the sweetest. Some people dislike sweet tea and others prefer to avoid sugar's 'empty' calories (refined carbohydrate that provides energy but no other nutrients). Those who give up sugary tea may find that inadvertently drinking it soon becomes anathema.

Decorating herb tea

Fresh flowers floating on hot or iced herb tea can look attractive. Suggestions include jasmine flowers, or borage or elderflower florets.

Storing tea or herb tea

Store dried tea or herb tea in an airtight 'caddy' made of dark glass, metal, porcelain or stoneware. Keep this away from sources of heat such as under-cupboard lighting, as heat encourages evaporation of a tea's essential oil. Tea keeps longer if refrigerated in an airtight container so it doesn't go mouldy. In a humid climate, consider storing tea in desiccant, oxygen-absorbing or vacuum-sealed packets (from certain stores or the Internet).

Check a tea has a 'best by' date. If it doesn't, write the purchase date on the container. Discard and replace any teas that are past their best-by dates, smell musty or have lost their scent.

Well-stored teas vary in 'keepability':

- Black teas generally stay good for at least one and sometimes two or three years; a few keep for decades.
- Green teas usually keep well for at least a year, although some begin to lose their flavour after six months. Gunpowder and other ball-shaped teas as well as large-leaf teas retain their fragrance for longer than looser-shaped, smaller-leaved or loose-leaf teas.

- Certain oolongs store well for decades.
- Loose-leaf *puerh* tea keeps for two to three years; *cheng puerh* for decades.
- Dried leaves and flowers for herb teas should keep for at least a year.
- Dried roots and rhizomes should keep for two to three years.
- Store fresh herbs in a brown paper or cotton bag.

Teapots

One made of stoneware or enamelled cast-iron is a good choice for black tea as it retains heat well. Porcelain, glass, enamelled tin and stainless steel lose heat faster, but are fine for green teas and herb teas. Pewter pots make a good cup of black tea, too.

Some teapots incorporate a removable infuser. Some people use a French press coffee-maker instead.

Asian-style teapots are usually small, holding enough tea for just one cup at a time.

Oolong tea is sometimes brewed in a special pot surrounded by an outer chamber of hot water to help the tea maintain its temperature.

Some people advocate simply rinsing a teapot after use, claiming that brown, tannin-rich deposits coating the inside add to the flavour of subsequent brews. If you do this, consider using different pots for strong, mild and scented teas.

You can wash your teapot if you prefer. Occasionally, you might want to clean it really well, by filling it with boiling hot water; adding a denture-cleaning tablet, tipping the pot so the solution runs into the spout; and leaving the full pot for an hour or more before rinsing.

Accessories

These include:

- **Ball infuser** (tea ball or tea egg) – a small perforated stainless-steel or plastic container, with handles, that sits in a cup or mug and contains the steeping tea leaves. It leaves very little space to expand and 'dance', so is best not used for premium whole-leaf teas.

- *Gaiwan* (or *zhong*) – a small cup with a lid and saucer, made of unglazed clay or thin porcelain, generally filled a quarter- to half-full with leaves, and useful for multiple steeping. The lid holds back the leaves when you pour the brew.

- **Mug infuser** – a plastic or stainless-steel mesh filter that sits in a cup or mug and contains the steeping leaves with plenty of room to expand and 'dance' as they hydrate. It's easy to use and quick to clean. You need one for each cup or mug of tea you are making at any one time.

- **Samovar** – a water-heater operated by electricity or with burning charcoal. Concentrated tea from a small teapot kept on top is diluted with hot water from the samovar's tap.

- **Tea caddy** – this wooden, metal or ceramic storage container ideally has an airtight lid.

- **Tea cosy** – better used only to keep a pot of *strained* tea warm.

- **Tea maker** – a machine that heats water and pours it over measured tea.

- **Tea scoop** – this is for measuring tea.

- **Teabag squeezer** – stainless-steel pincers for squeezing the remaining brew from a just-used teabag.

- **Teacup** – ideally one with relatively upright sides and made of pottery rather than thin china, so it keeps tea pleasantly hot for longer.

- **Tea strainer** – this strains a brew and is made of stainless steel or plastic.
- **Tea whisk** – made of bamboo, this mixes and froths Japanese powdered tea.

What to eat with teas

In the West, black tea is often accompanied by sweet foods such as biscuits, buns or cakes. In eastern Asia, green tea is often accompanied by savoury foods such as peanuts, and sometimes by biscuits or other sweet treats.

How much and how long?

General guidelines are:

- 4–6 cups of tea a day is a moderate intake, although many people happily and safely drink more. You need a minimum of 4 cups a day for optimal health benefit. The average Briton drinks about 3 cups a day.
- Up to 2–3 cups a day of everyday herb tea such as barley, chamomile, corn, dandelion, elderflower, hibiscus, peppermint or rooibos.
- Up to 1–2 cups a day of other herb tea to prevent an ailment or treat a chronic one; however, black cohosh, lemon balm and thyme teas are better not drunk on an ongoing daily basis.
- 3 cups a day of herb tea to treat an acute ailment.

Certain herb teas such as echinacea, ginseng and *Vitex agnus castus* may aid health most effectively if taken daily for several days, months or even years.

Cautions

Certain bioactive constituents can have adverse effects; most are short-lived and not serious, though. If you:

- Are pregnant or breastfeeding, or on medication, or have a chronic ailment, consult the list below.
- Have an oestrogen-sensitive cancer and are considering drinking a phytoestrogen-containing tea (barley, black cohosh, calendula, corn, dandelion, ginseng, red clover, nettle, rooibos, thyme, valerian, verbena and, probably, *Vitex agnus castus*), consult a doctor.
- Develop potentially serious allergic symptoms such as mouth swelling or breathing difficulty, get urgent medical help.
- Get dermatitis for the first time, consult a doctor.
- Have kidney stones, gallstones or period pain, avoid bitter-tasting teas.
- Have an inflamed gallbladder, painful gallstones, 'obstructive' jaundice or viral hepatitis (liver inflammation), avoid bile-stimulating teas (*see* page 86).

Each tea has particular safety notes:

Barley or roasted barley – can trigger an allergic reaction in a susceptible individual. Avoid it if you are gluten-sensitive (perhaps with coeliac disease). If on prescription medication, take it 1 hour before or 2 hours after the tea, as barley reduces the efficacy or increases the adverse effects of certain drugs. Consult a doctor first if on antidiabetic, blood-pressure-lowering or heart medication.

Black cohosh – avoid regular consumption for more than 6 months. It's best avoided during pregnancy or breastfeeding ('nursing').

Calendula – can trigger an allergic reaction in someone sensitive to ragweed. Avoid it during pregnancy or breastfeeding.

Chamomile – can trigger an allergic reaction in a susceptible person. It's best avoided during pregnancy as it can stimulate the womb.

Chickweed – is best avoided during pregnancy or breastfeeding as not enough safety data has been accumulated.

Cornsilk – aids fluid retention, but also flushes potassium from the body. So consult your doctor first if you are also taking diuretic medication.

Dandelion root – can trigger an allergic reaction in a susceptible person. Consult a doctor first if you have gallstones. It's best avoided during pregnancy or breastfeeding as safety data is unreliable.

Dong quai – can make skin more sensitive to sunlight, so use sunscreen when necessary. Consult a doctor first if on anticoagulants (blood thinners), medication for high blood pressure or an abnormal heart rhythm, selective-serotonin-reuptake-inhibitor anti-depressants or L-dopa medication (for Parkinson's disease); or if you have heavy periods or a hormone-sensitive cancer. It's probably best not taken long-term as its safrole might promote cancer. Avoid it during pregnancy or breastfeeding.

Echinacea – any immunity-boosting effect may gradually become less effective, so some experts suggest having a break every few weeks. Stop taking it before planned surgery as it can suppress immunity. Consult a doctor first if you have an autoimmune disorder. It is probably safe during pregnancy.

Elderflower – consult a doctor first if on anticancer chemotherapy or antidiabetes drugs. It's best avoided during pregnancy or breastfeeding as not enough safety data has been accumulated.

Ginseng – is often recommended for the over-40s – for men in particular, but not for premenopausal women. Some experts suggest that if young people take it, they should do so for only up to 3 weeks a month. Avoid other stimulants such as coffee and tea. Also, avoid it if you are anxious or depressed, or have an infection, an inflammatory condition or acute asthma. It can provoke unwanted oestrogenic effects. Consult your doctor if you are on anticoagulants (blood-thinners), antipsychotics, blood-pressure-lowering medication or steroids. Stop it at least 7 days before planned surgery to prevent low blood sugar and bleeding during or after the operation. Avoid it during pregnancy or breastfeeding.

Hibiscus – is relatively acidic, so avoid it if you are prone to acid reflux (heartburn). Also avoid it if you are taking the painkiller paracetamol (acetaminophen) as it can increase its adverse effects. It can trigger an allergic reaction in someone sensitive to the mallow family of plants. It's best avoided during pregnancy or breastfeeding. Also, avoid if you are trying to conceive as it can reduce fertility.

Lavender – safety information is incomplete, so drink only 1–2 cups a day for enjoyment, or to prevent ailments or treat chronic (long-lasting) ones; and only 3 cups a day to treat an acute ailment. Also, avoid it during pregnancy or breastfeeding. It can trigger an allergic reaction in a susceptible person. It can increase the effects (wanted and unwanted) of antidepressant and sedative medications; consult a doctor first if you are taking diazepam or lorazepam. Avoid it for 2 weeks before planned surgery as it can magnify the nervous-system dampening effect of anaesthesia or medication.

Lemon balm – daily use over a long time can depress thyroid function.

Avoid if you are on barbiturates as it can prolong their action. It's probably safe during pregnancy or breastfeeding.

Linden – consult a doctor first if you are on anticoagulants (blood thinners) or medication for high blood pressure, heart disease or lithium (for bipolar disease) as it can increase their effects. It's probably safe during pregnancy or breastfeeding, although research data is scant.

Nettle – consult a doctor if you are on medication, since it may interact with certain drugs such as anticoagulants (blood thinners) and certain other medications, including some of those for diabetes and high blood pressure. Avoid it during pregnancy or breastfeeding.

Passionflower – may trigger dizziness or sleepiness or, in a suscep-tible person, an allergic reaction. It can interact with certain drugs, including anticoagulants (blood thinners) and benzodiazepine tran-quillizers. Avoid it during pregnancy or breastfeeding.

Peppermint – avoid it if chilled by an upper respiratory infection or during gallstone pain. It's probably safe during pregnancy or breastfeeding.

Red clover – avoid it during pregnancy or breastfeeding. Also, avoid it for at least a week before planned surgery.

Rooibos – consult a doctor if you are on anticancer chemotherapy.

Rosehip – is possibly safe during pregnancy or breastfeeding, although not enough safety data has been accumulated.

Rosemary – is best avoided during pregnancy or breastfeeding.

Tea – experts suggest the average adult's all-source caffeine consump-tion (*see* page 57) should ideally be no more than 300mg a day or, during pregnancy and breastfeeding, 200mg a day. Note that 7–8 cups of average-strength tea, or 5 cups of very strong tea, provides 300mg caffeine. However, studies show no adverse effects from 6–9 average cups a day.

Much more might irritate the stomach and cause anxiety, twitchy muscles, a raised heart-rate, palpitation, insomnia (from tea drunk within 4 hours of trying to sleep), and, later, fatigue. Unusually, caffeine-sensitive individuals may have insomnia or a faster heartbeat after smaller amounts. At least 250mg caffeine in one sitting is needed for a diuretic effect. Caffeine temporarily raises blood pressure in those unused to it. Suddenly stopping regular consumption can cause headaches. Two large long-term studies found an association between high caffeine intake and precancerous or high-risk breast conditions in women.

Black tea reduces iron absorption by 60 per cent; green tea by 30 per cent. An intake of fewer than 8 cups a day is unlikely to harm iron status in healthy people whose diet is varied and balanced. But if you have iron-deficiency anaemia, it's wise to abstain during a meal and for the hour afterwards.

The caffeine and tannins in tea can also change the absorption or alter the effects of certain drugs. If you are on medication, check the patient information leaflet or ask your doctor to see if yours is one of them.

Black tea contains oxalates that encourage oxalate kidney stones in certain people. Longer steeping produces higher oxalate levels. But adding milk to tea discourages stones and can have other effects, too (*see* page 64).

Green tea makes the anticoagulant warfarin less effective.

Thyme – can trigger an allergic reaction in someone sensitive to plants in the mint family. Consult a doctor if you are on anticoagulants (blood thinners) as it can increase their action. Avoid it if you have heart disease or epilepsy. More than an occasional cup is probably best avoided in pregnancy as it can stimulate the womb.

Valerian – can add to the sedative effects of alcohol or drugs such as barbiturates and benzodiazepine tranquillizers. Consult a doctor first if you are taking these drugs or anti-convulsant drugs. Avoid it during pregnancy or breastfeeding.

Verbena – avoid regular large or therapeutic amounts. Avoid it during pregnancy (although it can be taken in labour to stimulate contractions) or breastfeeding.

Vitex agnus castus – avoid it if you are using oral contraception (the pill) or hormone replacement therapy, or are pregnant or breastfeeding.

Yarrow – can trigger an allergic reaction (such as contact dermatitis and photosensitive dermatitis triggered by sunlight), dizziness and headaches. Avoid it during pregnancy or breastfeeding.

Children and teas

Chamomile tea is considered generally safe in small amounts for babies older than six months. But if you are breastfeeding, note that liquids other than breast milk can reduce a breastfed baby's need for breast milk. Any resulting reduction in the frequency and length of feeds will reduce your milk supply.

For children over one year old, elderflower and peppermint teas, and 'true' tea, are considered generally safe in small amounts as occasional everyday drinks.

CHAPTER FIVE

Natural remedies

'True' tea and herb teas are popular folk remedies recommended in various healing systems, including ayurveda and traditional Chinese medicine. Scientific research increasingly supports their use.

Whole-leaf tea is richer in bioactive constituents than chopped, fragmented or powdered tea. Herbs are best processed just before use.

Your chosen brew should be appropriate for your ailment. It's a good idea to blend herbs, including one or more to treat your particular symptoms, along with a tonic herb to promote self-healing.

Using teas for common ailments

The most common way is to drink a tea (*see* page 75 for how often and how long). Elderly people need less. Children often refuse herb tea. If they are content to drink it, offer a small amount (for example, half the adult dose for a 12-year-old; a quarter for a 4-year-old).

You can also use a tea for a:
Bath – add a pint of the tea to the bathwater.

Compress – arthritis, backache, boils, muscle aching, infected wounds and ulcers respond better at first to a hot compress. Tension headaches and sprains do better at first with a cold one. Mucilage-rich herb teas (*see* page 44) make good hot compresses.

After a few days, it's possible to speed healing by alternating hot and cold compresses several times during a treatment session, ending with a cold one.

For a hot compress: soak a piece of cotton fabric or a cotton pad in the hot tea. When sufficiently cool, squeeze it out and apply it to the affected area. To keep it hot, either cover it with cling film, then a towel or hot-water bottle; or re-soak it in hot tea when necessary, then reapply.

For a cold compress: cool the tea first.

If necessary, secure it with a crêpe bandage.

Eyebath (eyecup) – one bought from a pharmacy or a small shallow dish. Before use, sterilize it by washing it in a dishwasher with a heated drying cycle or pour just-boiled water into it. Then let it stand for 1 minute.

Strain the tea then simmer it for 10 minutes to sterilize it; cool it to body temperature, then pour some into the eyebath. Leaning slightly backwards, pour a little into the affected eye.

Cover the remaining tea with cling film and refrigerate for later use. Next day, make a fresh supply.

Facial steam – put a pint of a just-made tea into a bowl on a table. Sit, leaning over the bowl, with a towel draped over your head and the bowl, for 5 minutes.

Footbath – fill a large bowl three-quarters with water, plus a pint (600ml) of a very strong tea. Use it hot or cold. Putting a cold compress on your forehead, while soaking your feet in a hot footbath, can be soothing for a feverish cold, cough or sore throat.

Another option is to soak your feet in a bowl of a hot tea for 2 minutes, then a bowl of cold tea for 2 minutes. Repeat several times.

Gargle – continue for at least 20 seconds and repeat 2–3 times a day.

Hair rinse – pour tea over your hair after shampooing.

Mouthwash – swill a tea around your mouth, then spit it out.

Poultice – discard the liquid from your chosen brew, let the wet leaves cool enough to be comfortable, then put them onto the affected area. Cover with a cotton pad followed by cling film. Mucilage-rich herb tea (*see* page 44) makes a good poultice.

Steam inhalation – as for 'Facial steam', but inhale deeply.

Medicinal actions of teas

Traditional uses and/or scientific studies indicate various actions. The underlined teas have moderately strong or strong effects.

Adaptogenic (a nervous-system 'tonic' that increases resistance to stress, probably by boosting or reducing – depending on need – adrenal hormones such as adrenaline): ginseng, rooibos.

Analgesic (relieves pain): black cohosh, calendula, chamomile, chickweed, dandelion, dong quai, echinacea, elderlflower, lavender, passionflower, peppermint, rosemary, tea, thyme, valerian.

Antiallergic: chamomile, echinacea, lemon balm, nettle, tea.

Antibacterial: barley, calendula, chamomile, chickweed, dandelion, dong quai, echinacea, elderflower, hibiscus, lavender, lemon balm, linden, nettle, peppermint, red clover, rosehip, rosemary, tea (especially green), thyme, valerian.

Anticancer: barley, black cohosh, calendula, chickweed, corn, dandelion, dong quai, echinacea, elderflower, ginseng, hibiscus, lavender, peppermint, red clover, rooibos, rosehip, rosemary, tea, valerian.

Anticoagulant (thins blood): roasted barley, chamomile, dong quai, ginseng, nettle, red clover, tea (especially green).

Anticonvulsant: chamomile, lavender, linden, passionflower, rosemary, valerian (if convulsions are provoked by poor sleep), verbena.

Antidepressant: black cohosh, calendula, chamomile, dandelion, dong quai, elderflower, ginseng, lavender, lemon balm, linden, nettle, passionflower, peppermint, red clover, rooibos, rosehip, rosemary, tea (especially green) and valerian.

Antifungal: calendula, chamomile, dandelion, dong quai, echinacea, hibiscus, lavender, peppermint, rosemary, tea, thyme.

Antihistamine: chamomile, dong quai, lemon balm, nettle.

Anti-inflammatory: black cohosh, calendula, chamomile, chickweed, cornsilk, dandelion, dong quai, echinacea, elderflower, ginseng, hibiscus, lavender, lemon balm, linden, nettle, peppermint, red clover, rooibos, rosehip, rosemary, red clover, tea.

Antioxidant: barley, calendula, chickweed, dandelion, echinacea, lavender, lemon balm, linden, nettle, peppermint, rooibos, rosehip, rosemary, tea (especially green), thyme, verbena.

Antispasmodic (relaxes tense skeletal muscle or tenses 'smooth' muscle in blood vessels, breathing passages, gut or womb): black cohosh, calendula, chamomile, dong quai, echinacea, elderflower, hibiscus, lavender, lemon balm, linden, nettle, passionflower, peppermint, red clover, rosemary, tea, thyme, valerian, verbena, *Vitex agnus castus*.

Antiviral: calendula, chamomile, dandelion, dong quai, echinacea, lemon balm, peppermint, rooibos, rosehip, tea (especially green), thyme.

Astringent (reduces bleeding and inflammation of skin and mucus production by mucous membrane): calendula, chickweed, dandelion, echinacea, elderflower, hibiscus, linden, nettle, peppermint, rooibos, rosehip, rosemary, tea, thyme, verbena.

Bile-stimulating (boosts bile production or flow): the 'bitters' or 'bitter principles' – calendula, dandelion, dong quai, lavender, lemon balm, linden, peppermint, nettle, rosemary, verbena.

Bitter-tasting (*see* page 41): barley, black cohosh, calendula, chamomile, dandelion, dong quai, ginseng, hibiscus, nettle, rooibos, rosehip, rosemary, thyme, verbena.

Blood-cell-boosting: dong quai, echinacea.

Blood-fat-lowering: cornsilk, dandelion, elderflower, ginseng, rooibos, tea.

Blood-pressure-lowering: black cohosh, dong quai, ginseng, hibiscus, linden, nettle, passionflower, tea, valerian, verbena; also antispasmodic, diuretic and relaxant teas.

Blood-sugar-lowering: black cohosh, calendula, cornsilk, dandelion, dong quai, elderflower, ginseng, hibiscus, nettle, rosemary, tea.

Cholesterol-lowering: roasted barley, black cohosh, cornsilk, dandelion, dong quai, elderflower, ginseng, hibiscus, lavender, linden, rosehip, tea, thyme.

Decongestant: dandelion, elderflower, nettle, peppermint, tea, thyme.

Demulcent (soothes and protects mucous membranes, so can, for example, reduce colic, coughs and diarrhoea): barley, calendula, chickweed, cornsilk.

Digestive (boosts appetite and aids digestion – possibly by boosting saliva and digestive enzymes): calendula, chamomile, cinnamon (boosts trypsin), dandelion (leaf/root), dong quai, echinacea, elderflower, lavender, lemon balm, linden, passionflower, peppermint, rosehip, rosemary, tea, thyme, verbena (*see* also 'Bile-stimulating').

Diuretic (increases urine production, so reducing blood pressure and weight): black cohosh, calendula, chamomile, chickweed, cornsilk, dandelion, dong quai, elderflower, hibiscus, linden, nettle, peppermint, red clover, rooibos, rosehip, rosemary, tea, thyme, valerian.

Emollient (soothes and protects inflamed skin): barley, calendula, chickweed, cornsilk.

Expectorant (increases and dilutes bronchial secretions, making them easier to cough up): chickweed, dong quai, elderflower, hibiscus, linden, nettle, peppermint, red clover, thyme, valerian, verbena.

Hormone-balancing:

   Adrenaline (epinephrine) and **noradrenaline** (norepinephrine) – *see* 'Neurotransmitters'.

   Cortisol (hydrocortisone) – raises blood sugar and reduces immune reactions. Echinacea boosts its production.

   Oestrogens – phytoestrogens (in barley, black cohosh, calendula, corn, dandelion, ginseng, nettle, red clover, rooibos, tea thyme, valerian, verbena and, probably, *Vitex agnus castus*) help balance high or low levels. Dandelion can reduce high oestrogen by aiding its breakdown. *Vitex agnus castus* reduces oestrogen production (by decreasing follicle-stimulating hormone).

Progesterone – dandelion enhances its action. *Vitex agnus castus* boosts it (by encouraging ovulation and by boosting dopamine (*see* 'Neurotransmitter-action boosting'), thus inhibiting the hormone prolactin.

Testosterone – ginseng can increase it.

Thyroid hormones – lemon balm may lower high levels. But it may also improve mild thyroid underactivity from an autoimmune disorder (possibly thanks to its selenium).

Immunity-boosting: calendula, dandelion, dong quai, echinacea, elderflower, ginseng, hibiscus, peppermint, rosehip, tea (especially green); also circulation-boosting herbs (which boost white-cell production).

Laxative (bowel-stimulating): chickweed, dandelion, dong quai, elderflower, linden, rosehip, verbena.

Neurotransmitter (nerve-message-carrier)-action-boosting: this may result from reduced breakdown, or activation of their cell receptors.

Acetylcholine – this 'rest-and-digest' neurotransmitter slows the heart; encourages stomach and bowel movements; dilates blood vessels (lowering blood pressure like calcium-channel-blocker drugs); improves memory and concentration and therefore the speed and accuracy of learning; and affects mood and skeletal-muscle movement. These actions are increased by chamomile, dong quai, ginseng, nettle, lemon balm, peppermint, rosemary, tea and valerian.

Adrenaline and noradrenaline – are also hormones. Adrenaline increases heart rate, breathing rate, blood sugar, blood pressure and blood flow to muscles; and sharpens senses. Ginseng and tea increase these actions. Noradrenaline increases heart rate and blood pressure, widens airways and directs more blood to essential organs, and tea increases these actions (*see* also 'General').

Cannabinoids – the actions of those that reduce inflammation and pain and, perhaps, prostate cancer and osteoporosis, are increased by alkylamides (in echinacea) and β-caryophyllene (in dong quai, echinacea, lavender, lemon balm, rosemary and *Vitex agnus castus*). The actions of those that encourage the feeling of well-being are increased by epigallocatechin (in tea, especially green tea).

Dopamine – this produces satisfaction and aids fine-movement control; its actions are increased by tea and *Vitex agnus castus*.

Gamma-aminobutyric acid (GABA) – the action of this calming and relaxing neurotransmitter is increased by lavender, lemon balm, passionflower, tea, thyme and valerian. (Benzodiazepine tranquillizers also work this way.)

Monoamine-oxidase inhibitors – these inhibit monoamine oxidase, the enzyme that breaks down adrenaline, dopamine, melatonin, noradrenaline and serotonin, thereby increasing their action. This could reduce depression or otherwise stabilise mood. (Monoamine-oxidase-inhibitor medications work in the same way.)

They include:

- Anthocyanins (in rosehip).
- Epicatechin (in tea).
- Certain flavonoids: apigenin (in chickweed, lemon balm,

passionflower, rosemary and thyme); kaempferol (in calendula, chickweed, elderflower, lemon balm, linden, nettle, passionflower, rosemary, tea and *Vitex agnus castus*); and quercetin (in calendula, chamomile, elder-flower, lemon balm, linden, nettle, passionflower, rooibos, rosehip, rosemary, tea and valerian).

- Harman-group alkaloids (in barley, cornsilk and passionflower).
- Quercetin (in calendula, chamomile, elderflower, lemon balm, linden, nettle, passionflower, rooibos, rosehip, rosemary, tea and valerian) which can be an antidepressant.
- Scopoletin (in dong quai).

Serotonin – the actions of this 'feel-good' neurotransmitter are boosted by black cohosh, dandelion, ginseng, peppermint, red clover, tea and valerian.

Sedating (calms body *and* mind): black cohosh, chamomile, dandelion, dong quai, ginseng (which, because of its adaptogenic properties, can instead be stimulating, if necessary), lavender, lemon balm, linden, peppermint, red clover, rooibos, thyme, valerian, verbena.

Sleep-inducing (hypnotic): chamomile, dandelion, lavender, linden, passionflower, valerian, verbena.

Stimulating (stimulates nerves): dong quai, echinacea, elderflower, ginseng (which, because of its adaptogenic properties, can instead be sedating, if necessary), linden, peppermint, rosehip, rosemary, tea, thyme.

Tonic ('normalises' the body's self-healing; herbs traditionally called 'alteratives', which aid healing by altering metabolism in unspecified ways, are included here): chickweed, rooibos and, for the following systems:

- Cardiovascular: linden.
- Digestive: chamomile, dandelion, nettle.
- Hormonal: phytoestrogens, *Vitex agnus castus*.
- Liver: bitter-tasting herbs.
- Urinary: cornsilk, nettle.
- Nervous system: ginseng, red clover, verbena.
- Musculoskeletal: black cohosh, nettle.
- Reproductive: black cohosh.
- Respiratory: echinacea.
- Skin: echinacea, nettle, red clover.

Tranquillizing (eases anxiety): black cohosh, chamomile, lavender, lemon balm, linden, passionflower, tea, thyme, valerian, verbena, *Vitex agnus castus*.

Warming teas contain substances that:

- Boost metabolism and therefore increase heat production. This is partly thanks to certain alkaloids and aromatics, for example, in chickweed, dandelion, hibiscus and tea.
- Speed the heart rate and therefore boost the circulation. This is mostly thanks to certain alkaloids, glycosides and phenolic compounds, for example, in nettle, rosemary and thyme.
- Dilate small arteries and veins (*see* 'Antispasmodic').

Wind/gas-expelling (carminative): chamomile, echinacea, dong quai, elderflower, lavender, lemon balm, linden, nettle, peppermint, rooibos, rosemary, thyme, valerian.

Wound healing (vulnerary, stimulating new cell growth): calendula, chamomile, echinacea, linden, red clover, rosemary, thyme.

Traditional uses and scientific backing of tea and herb teas

Scientific studies back up many of the traditional medicinal uses of tea and herb teas. Although much of the research is early, the findings are nonetheless exciting.

'True' tea is traditionally used *as a drink* – for acne; allergy; anxiety; asthma; atherosclerosis; athlete's foot; certain cancers; colds; coughs; depression; diarrhoea; eczema; fatigue; fever; flu; fluid retention; high cholesterol; indigestion; insomnia; migraine; muscle aching; obesity; shingles; tooth decay; and wounds.

In particular:

Black tea is used for diarrhoea, hangovers and, *externally*, for athlete's foot (as a footbath); cold sores (as a wash); shingles (as a compress or wash); tooth decay (as a mouthwash); and wounds (as a compress or poultice).

Green tea is used for arthritis; bad breath; diabetes; infection; inflammatory bowel disease; obesity; poor immunity; and, *externally*, used for conjunctivitis and sties (as an eyebath). It is also used to aid longevity.

Scientific studies show or suggest that 'true' tea is a potent antioxidant; discourages allergy; improves 'atopic' eczema; reduces high cholesterol, fats and blood pressure (3 cups a day of black tea reduce this by 2–3 points); discourages flu and herpes (5 cups a day raise virus-fighting interferon tenfold); protects against heart attacks (3 cups a day reduce the risk by 11 per cent) and strokes; slows memory loss and cognitive decline; discourages certain cancers and type-2 diabetes; and may improve bone strength.

In particular, its:

Caffeine and **theanine** boost concentration and mental relaxation; caffeine may discourage Parkinson's disease.

Caffeine, **catechins** and **theanine** promote fat loss (by inhibiting enzymes that digest fats), specifically, the loss of visceral fat, the 'belly fat' highly associated with an increased risk of type-2 diabetes and metabolic syndrome.

Catechins may discourage Alzheimer's disease, eye diseases (such as glaucoma), candida and, perhaps, osteoporosis.

Epigallocatechin gallate's anti-inflammatory effects inhibit the excessive production of the COX-2 enzyme that encourages arthritis and cancer. It may also reduce weight by helping to convert calories into muscle, not fat, by prolonging the metabolism-boosting action of noradrenaline (norepinephrine), and by reducing appetite.* It also reduces brain damage after a stroke.*

Fluroride discourages tooth decay.

Tannins might help diarrhoea and heavy periods.

Theophylline widens airways and arteries and reduces cholesterol.*

Also, for green tea: 1 cup is more antioxidant than a serving of broccoli, carrots, spinach or strawberries. It also helps prevent abnormal blood clots. And it may discourage 'all-cause death'.*

(* Research done in humans)

A–Z of common ailments

This details which teas can help common health problems. The suggestions should not replace medical diagnosis and therapy. Consult a doctor or pharmacist before taking large amounts of any tea. Refer to page 84 for which teas have which medicinal properties and check 'Cautions' on page 76.

Acne

Antibacterial, anti-inflammatory and astringent teas may help. In particular, *Vitex agnus castus* may be useful.

Action: Include these teas in your diet.

Bathe affected skin twice a day with one of them.

Alzheimer's disease

Anti-inflammatory and antioxidant teas may help. Alzheimer's is associated with damage to the brain's acetylcholine-producing system. The body uses choline to make acetylcholine; so choline-containing teas (*see* page 42) might help. In addition, lemon balm tea may reduce agitation associated with Alzheimer's.

Action: Include these teas in your diet.

Anaemia

If you have iron-deficiency anaemia, dandelion and nettle teas offer iron, and dong-quai tea can boost blood-cell production.

Action: Include these teas in your diet.

Anxiety

Antispasmodic and tranquillizing teas may help. In particular, try passionflower (since research suggests this may relieve anxiety faster, and as effectively, as the antianxiety drug oxazepam). Lavender tea may help by making the relaxing neurotransmitter GABA (*see* page 89) more efficient. Note that even just inhaling the fragrance of a cup of lavender tea can reduce anxiety.

Action: Include these teas in your diet. Passionflower and valerian could be a useful blend.

Also inhale the fragrance of the steam from any of these hot teas, especially lavender.

Arthritis

Analgesic, anti-inflammatory, antioxidant and antispasmodic teas may help. In particular, note that rosehip tea may reduce pain and boost joint mobility in people with osteoarthritis. Also, nettle tea can reduce the need for medication for osteoarthritis.

Action: Include these teas in your diet.

Apply a compress or a poultice containing one of them over the affected joint.

Asthma

Antiallergic, antihistamine, anti-inflammatory, antioxidant and anti-spasmodic teas may help.

Action: Include these teas in your diet.

Also inhale steam from one of them once or twice a day.

Atherosclerosis

Anti-inflammatory, antioxidant, anticoagulant, cholesterol-lowering and blood-sugar-lowering teas may help this narrowing and stiffening of the arteries.

Action: Include these teas in your diet.

Autoimmune diseases

Tea's catechins may reduce the raised levels of autoantibodies associated with diseases such as lupus.

Action: Include tea in your diet.

Bad breath

Antibacterial teas may help, in particular barley or roasted barley tea.

Action: Use them as a mouthwash.

Bruises

Rosehip and rosemary teas may help.

Action: Include these teas in your diet.

Also apply them in a compress or a poultice to the bruised area.

Cancer

Early research suggests that certain constituents of teas may aid prevention and/or treatment via their effects on certain enzymes, cell-signalling pathways and genes as these can modify cancer-cell multiplication, the formation of new blood vessels to support cancer growth and cancer-cell apoptosis ('cell suicide'). Discouraging apoptosis is thought to be the most common beneficial effect. However, such constituents are present in teas mostly in very small quantities, and any benefits in humans are, as yet, largely unproven.

They include:

Alkylamides (in echinacea); antibacterial substances (*see* page 84); β-elemene [rnds] (in ginseng); **carnosol** (in rosemary); **antioxidants** (*see* page 85); β-caryophyllene (in dong quai, echinacea, lavender, lemon balm, rosemary and *Vitex agnus castus*); chlorophyll (in nettle and peppermint); ellagic acid (in rosehip); farnesol (in linden); epicatechin and **epigallocatechin gallate** (in tea); **ginsenosides** (in ginseng); limonene (in dong quai, peppermint, rosemary and verbena); **perillyl alcohol** (in lavender); flavonoids such as **quercetin** (in calendula, chamomile, elderflower, lemon balm, linden, nettle, passionflower, rooibos, rosehip, rosemary, tea and valerian); **quninones** (in chickweed, nettle, rosemary and verbena); various phenolic compounds; **salicylates** (*see* page 49); **selenium** (in barley); **trigonelline** (in barley and corn); and **valepotriates** (in valerian and verbena).

Also:

- **β-sitosterol** (in chickweed, corn, dandelion, dong quai, elderflower, nettle and red clover) inhibits the growth of oestrogen-receptor-positive *and* -negative breast cancer cells. (When combined with the medication tamoxifen, the inhibition of oestrogen-receptor-positive cells is greater.)
- **Phytoestrogens** (*see* page 45) are weaker than own oestrogens, so may help prevent 'oestrogen-receptor positive' (therefore oestrogen-sensitive) cancers encouraged by high levels of a person's own oestrogen. However, they could reduce the beneficial effect of oestrogen-lowering medication for an existing oestrogen-sensitive cancer.
- **Ursolic acid** (in elderflower, lavender, lemon balm,

peppermint, rosemary, thyme and verbena) enhances chemotherapy for multiple myeloma.

Very early evidence suggests that more research is warranted in case these teas might prove to help prevent or treat the following cancers:

- **Bladder**: tea
- **Bowel** – barley, calendula, chamomile, corn, elderflower, lavender, lemon balm, linden, nettle, passionflower, peppermint, rooibos, rosehip, rosemary, tea, valerian.
- **Brain**: dong quai, lavender, green tea.
- **Breast**: calendula, chamomile, cornsilk, dandelion leaf, dong quai, elderflower, ginseng, tea, lavender, lemon balm, linden, nettle, passionflower, red clover, rooibos, rosehip, rosemary, green tea, valerian.
- **Cervix**: barley, calendula, corn, green tea.
- **Fibrosarcoma**: calendula.
- **Head and neck**: calendula.
- **Leukaemia**: barley, calendula, corn, dandelion root, echinacea, green tea, nettle, rosemary, *Vitex agnus castus*.
- **Liver**: barley, calendula, corn, green tea, nettle, peppermint, rosemary.
- **Lung**: calendula, ginseng.
- **Lymphoma** (non-Hodgkin's): green tea.
- **Melanoma**: calendula, dandelion root, nettle, peppermint, rosemary, green tea.
- **Multiple myeloma**: elderflower, lavender, lemon balm, peppermint, rosemary, thyme, verbena.
- **Mouth**: tea.
- **Oesophagus** (gullet): green tea.
- **Ovary**: tea.

- **Pancreas**: calendula, lavender, tea.
- **Prostate**: barley, calendula, chamomile, dandelion, elderflower, ginseng, lavender, lemon balm, linden, nettle, passionflower, rooibos, rosehip, rosemary, green tea, valerian, *Vitex agnus castus*.
- **Stomach**: calendula, ginseng, rosemary, tea.
- **Womb**: green tea.

Action: in case they help prevent cancer, consider drinking the apparently appropriate teas.

Consult your doctor before taking any tea as a possible treatment, since certain teas make particular anticancer medications less effective, contain phytoestrogens better avoided with oestrogen-sensitive cancers, or encourage unwanted weight loss.

Cold sores (canker sores)
Anti-viral teas can help.

Action: Include these teas in your diet.

Also apply them frequently as a wash.

Colds, sore throats, sinusitis and flu
Astringent, antibacterial, anti-inflammatory, antiviral and decongestant teas may help. If you are feverish, consider diaphoretic (cooling) teas.

Action: Include these teas in your diet.

Also do an inhalation of the steam from them several times a day.

Conjunctivitis

Antibacterial, anti-inflammatory, antiviral and immunity-boosting teas may help.

Action: Include these teas in your diet.

Also use calendula, chamomile, chickweed, elderflower, rosemary or thyme tea in an eyebath.

Constipation

Try laxative teas, antianxiety teas (for constipation associated with stress) and teas rich in prebiotics (*see* page 42).

Action: Include these teas in your diet.

Cough

For a dry cough, anti-inflammatory, antioxidant, antiviral and demulcent teas can help.

For a productive cough, try antibacterial, anti-inflammatory, antioxidant, astringent, decongestant and expectorant ones.

Action: Include these teas in your diet.

Also do inhalations of the steam from one of them several times a day.

Cramp

Circulation-boosting and muscle-relaxing teas may help.

Action: Include these teas in your diet.

Cystitis

Antibacterial and anti-inflammatory teas may help.

Action: include these teas in your diet.

Dandruff (*see* 'Infection', page 104)

Depression

Antidepressant teas may help.

Action: Include these teas in your diet.

Also try inhaling the scent from lavender, lemon balm or rosehip tea every 2 hours or so.

Diabetes

Anti-inflammatory and blood-sugar-lowering teas may help. If you prefer sweet teas, drink those that are naturally sweet (*see* page 50) and, therefore, require no sweetening with sugar.

Action: Include these teas in your diet.

Diarrhoea

Anti-inflammatory, antioxidant, antibacterial, antispasmodic, antiviral, astringent and demulcent teas may help.

Action: Include these teas in your diet.

Eczema

Antiallergic, antihistamine, anti-inflammatory, antioxidant and astringent teas may help, as may coumarin-containing ones (*see* page 43).

Also for eczema over varicose veins, try circulation-boosting teas.

Action: Include these teas in your diet.

In addition, use these teas, and emollient teas, in a bath or in a compress, poultice or wash for the affected skin.

Fatigue

Warming and tonic teas may be invigorating. Rosehip tea may help as well.

Action: Include these teas in your diet.

Also try inhaling the scent of linden or rosemary teas as this can have an energising effect.

Fertility problems

Barley and dong quai teas may help male infertility. *Vitex agnus castus* can encourage ovulation.

Action: Include one or more of these teas in your diet for several months.

If hormone tests in the second half of your menstrual cycle reveal low progesterone (implying ovulation hasn't occurred), consider taking *Vitex agnus castus* each morning, starting on the first day of a period.

Fever

An antibacterial or antiviral tea can help fever resulting from infection, while diaphoretic teas are cooling.

Action: Include these teas in your diet.

Fibromyalgia

Anti-inflammatory, antispasmodic and diuretic teas may help.

Action: Include these teas in your diet.

Also put them in your bathtub water.

Fluid retention

Circulation-boosting (*see* 'Warming') and diuretic teas can help. Note that unlike many diuretic drugs, dandelion tea replaces the potassium lost from the blood as more urine is produced.

Action: Include these teas in your diet.

Gingivitis

Antibacterial and anti-inflammatory teas can help.

Action: Include these teas in your diet.

Headache and migraine

Analgesic teas may help: in particular, those containing salicylates (*see* page 49).

Also use anti-inflammatory and antispasmodic teas.

Action: Include these teas in your diet.

Apply a compress made with one of them, hot or cold according to what you find works best.

Heart disease (*see* 'Atherosclerosis')

High blood pressure

Anti-inflammatory, antioxidant, antispasmodic, blood-pressure-lowering, choline-containing (*see* page 42), diuretic and relaxing teas may help. If appropriate, add cholesterol-lowering and diuretic teas. In particular, try hibiscus tea: in one study, drinking 3 cups a day for 6 weeks reduced high blood pressure by 13 points! This was presumably because of its diuretic effect and its anthocyanins acting like blood-pressure drugs called angiotensin-converting enzyme (ACE) inhibitors. Rooibos tea can also act like an ACE-inhibitor drug.

Note that even just inhaling the fragrance of a cup of lavender tea can reduce high blood pressure.

Action: Include these teas in your diet.

High cholesterol

Antioxidant and cholesterol-lowering teas should help, as should teas rich in β-sitosterol (which may reduce fat absorption from the gut).

Action: Include these teas in your diet.

Indigestion

Antispasmodic, bitter, digestive and choline-containing teas may help. In particular, try peppermint.

Action: Include these teas in your diet.

Infection

Choose between antibacterial, antifungal and antiviral teas, depending on the likely infecting agent. Anti-inflammatory and astringent teas may help, too.

Action: Include these in your diet.
Also:

- For a boil, apply a compress or poultice made with an antibacterial tea.
- For a fungal skin infection, use a wash or bath of an antifungal tea.
- For dandruff, after washing your hair, apply a hair rinse of an antifungal tea mixed with 1 tablespoon of cider vinegar.

Irritable bowel

Anti-inflammatory, antispasmodic and digestive teas may help. In particular, try chamomile and peppermint teas.

Action: Include these teas in your diet.

Insomnia

Antianxiety (*see* page 95), sedative and acetylcholine-boosting teas may help. In particular, try valerian.

Action: Drink these teas with your evening meal.

Low sex drive

Teas that may help are ginseng (for men) and *Vitex agnus castus* (for women). Black cohosh, dong quai, hibiscus, red clover and rosehip teas are also reputedly useful.

Action: Include these teas in your diet.
    Inhale the fragrance of the steam from rosehip tea.

Menopause problems

Several herbal teas are traditionally used, including phytoestrogen-containing teas, as well as dong quai, passionflower and *Vitex agnus castus*. Early research is not very encouraging, though: the results for black cohosh are mixed, there is no convincing evidence for red clover and little for or against other commonly used herbs.

Action: Consider including these teas in your diet.

Muscle-aching

Analgesic, anti-inflammatory and antispasmodic teas may help.

Action: Include these teas in your diet.

Also use one or more of them in a compress, poultice or in your bathwater.

Neuralgia

Analgesic teas may be useful, as may, depending on the cause, antibacterial, anti-inflammatory, antispasmodic and antiviral teas.

Action: Include these teas in your diet.

Also apply them in a compress to or wash the affected area.

Obesity

Metabolism-boosting teas may help (*see* 'Warming', page 91). Also, try appetite-reducing teas such as chickweed, dandelion, nettle, peppermint (even the scent of which reduces appetite) and red clover. Teas rich in β-sitosterol can reduce fat absorption from the gut. And the phaseolamin in hibiscus tea could help by reducing starch absorption from the gut. Also, ginseng can promote weight loss.

Action: Include these teas in your diet.

Pain

Analgesic teas (*see* page 84) can help.

Action: Include these teas in your diet.

Period problems

• *Heavy periods*: astringent, phytoestrogen-containing and tannin-containing teas (*see* page 45) may help. In particular, try

Vitex agnus castus.

- *Period pain*: analgesic and antispasmodic teas may help. Black cohosh or *Vitex agnus castus* is particularly worth including.
- *Premenstrual syndrome*: try *Vitex agnus castus*.
- *Scanty periods*: phytoestrogen-containing teas may help, as may rosemary (though why isn't clear) and *Vitex agnus castus*.

Action: Include the appropriate teas in your diet.

Poor circulation

Warming teas may help.

Action: Include these teas in your diet.

Poor immunity

Immunity-enhancing, circulation-boosting (*see* 'Warming', page 91) and tonic teas may help. Rooibos tea, for example, enhances immunity by boosting natural body substances called interleukins.

Action: Include these teas in your diet.

Poor memory

Circulation-boosting teas may help, as may teas containing ferulic acid (*see* page 36) or rutin (*see* page 49) and ginseng.

Action: Include these teas in your diet.

Premature ageing

Antioxidant teas may help. Rosemary tea and green tea are traditionally associated with longevity.

Action: Include these teas in your diet.

Psoriasis

Anti-inflammatory teas may help, as may coumarin-containing ones (*see* page 43).

Action: Include these teas in your diet.

Use these teas and emollient teas as a wash or in a bath, or apply them to affected patches of skin in a compress or poultice.

Sprains

Locally applied calendula, lavender, nettle or rosemary teas may help.

Action: Apply one or more of them in a compress or a poultice.

Tooth decay

Analgesic and antibacterial teas may help. Barley and corn teas, and tea, help prevent decay.

Action: Include these teas in your diet.

Use antibacterial teas and green tea as a mouthwash after eating.

Varicose veins

Rutin-containing teas (*see* page 49) may help; also, if the veins are inflamed, use anti-inflammatory teas.

Action: Include these teas in your diet.

Also apply them in a compress or a poultice.

Wind

Digestive and wind-reducing teas should help.

Action: Include these teas in your diet.

Wounds and sores

Astringent, antibacterial, anti-inflammatory, antiviral, blood-vessel-relaxing, demulcent and wound-healing teas may help.

Action: Include these teas in your diet.

Bathe affected skin with one of them or apply a tea-soaked compress.

CHAPTER SIX

You and your home

Certain teas and herb teas can help you nurture and beautify your skin and hair, and some can be useful around the home.

Beauty care

The bioactive constituents in teas and herb teas can have beneficial effects on skin and hair when the tea is either drunk or applied to the skin. Indeed, many of these constituents are important ingredients of certain commercially made beauty products.

When applied to the skin, some are:

Anti-inflammatory – antioxidants can soothe skin.

Astringent – caffeine and tannins reduce oiliness, help close pores and tighten skin.

Emollient – allantoin and mucilage help hydrate, protect and soothe skin.

Moisturising and exfoliating – allantoin and alpha-hydroxy acids (AHAs) can moisturise and therefore smooth and soften cracked, dry, flaking or hard skin.

TABLE 8: SKIN-FRIENDLY CONSTITUENTS OF SELECTED TEAS

	AHAs	Allantoin	Caffeine or tannin	Mucilage	Anti-bacterials	Diosmin, hesperidin or rutin
Calendula				●	●	●
Chamomile			●		●	●
Chickweed				●	●	●
Cornsilk		●	●			
Dandelion			●	●	●	
Elderflower			●	●	●	●
Hibiscus	●				●	
Lavender			●		●	
Linden			●	●		●
Nettle			●	●	●	●
Passion flower						●
Peppermint			●		●	●
Rooibos	●					●
Rosehip	●			●	●	●
Rosemary			●		●	●
Tea	●		●		●	●
Thyme			●		●	
Verbena			●	●		

Certain others:

Improve photo-aged skin – allantoin promotes new-cell growth.
Antioxidants help protect against sun damage and wrinkles. Certain
AHAs, including citric acid, increase the production of collagen (a
connective tissue) and certain polysaccharides, making skin thicker
and more supple.

Discourage 'broken veins' – certain flavonoid pigments such as
hesperidin and rutin strengthen blood-vessel walls, so may shrink
the dilated capillaries (tiny blood vessels) sometimes called
'broken veins'.

All teas contain antioxidants. This table of other skin-friendly
bioactive constituents will help you choose the most appropriate teas
for your skin:

For everyday skin-care

Use your chosen tea warm or cool. Either apply it as a 'splash' while
leaning over the wash basin or apply it with a cotton pad. Then let
your skin dry naturally.

For example, if you have:

- **Oily skin**: cleanse and tone with a tea that contains an
  astringent but no mucilage – such as chamomile, cornsilk,
  lavender, rosemary, tea or thyme.
- **Dry skin**: cleanse and moisturise with a tea containing mucilage
  but free from astringents and AHAs – such as calendula,
  chickweed, passionflower or rooibos.
- **Mature skin**: cleanse and moisturise with a tea that contains
  mucilage and/or blood-vessel-strengtheners but free from
  astringents and AHAs – such as calendula, chickweed or
  passionflower. As long as your skin isn't dry, cornsilk is a good
  choice because it contains allantoin.

For fine lines around the eyes

Note that used teabags containing one of the teas listed above for mature skin can help smooth out these 'laughter lines'. Simply lie down, rest the teabag over your closed eyes for 10–15 minutes and relax.

For more intensive skin-care

Each week use one of these:

- **Face mask**: put 2 tablespoons of bran (from a health food shop) into a bowl and 1 teaspoon of runny honey. Stir in 3 tablespoons of a tea appropriate to your skin type. Apply the mixture to your face, leave it on for 10 minutes, then rinse it off with warm water.
- **Facial steam** (*see* page 83).

For your bath (bathtub)

Choose a 'bath tea' according to whether you would like it to help you relax (chamomile, chickweed, lavender, linden, passionflower and verbena) or be invigorating (elderflower, linden, peppermint, rosehip, tea and thyme). Ideally, choose a tea that's appropriate for your skin type.

For hair care

Use herb teas to:

- **Darken greying hair** – 12 hours before you need it, steep 3 rosemary teabags in 1 cup of boiling water. Add 2 tablespoons of dried rosemary (or 6 of fresh). Let it stand for 12 hours, then strain it. After shampooing, pour it through your hair. Don't rinse it out with water, but simply dry your hair with an old towel. This has only a very slightly darkening effect, but repeating it will produce some further darkening.
- **Enhance hair growth** – after shampooing, apply linden tea and wait for 5 minutes before rinsing.

- **Give shine to natural highlights in blonde hair** – after shampooing, apply calendula or chamomile tea and wait for 5 minutes before rinsing.
- **Reduce hair loss** – for general loss, calendula, nettle, rosemary and thyme teas may help. For male-pattern loss (from oversensitivity to the hormone dihydrotestosterone in men and women), chickweed, corn, dandelion, dong quai, elderflower and red clover teas (thanks to their sterols), and tea (thanks to its caffeine and epigallocatechin gallate), may help. After shampooing, apply one of them and wait 5 minutes before rinsing. Also, include these teas in your diet.
- **Help dry hair shine** – after shampooing, rinse with warm tea, then dry your hair with an old towel.
- **Scent hair** – after shampooing, rinse with rosemary tea.

Deodorant

After washing and drying your armpits, smooth on some linden tea and let your skin dry naturally. Linden tea contains an aromatic called farnesol which has antibacterial activity and is included in some commercially produced deodorants. The amount of farnesol in linden tea is small, but may be helpful.

Uses in the home

Tea or herb tea can:
- **Absorb unwanted smells** – keep unused teabags in an airtight container so you can put them in a shallow dish to absorb formaldehyde from fresh paint or glue; newly cut particle-board, plywood or pressed-wood products; and urea-formaldehyde-

foam insulation. Wet tea leaves help remove the smell of fish from a pan.

- **Clean wood furniture and floors** – put 2 black-tea teabags into a bowl, add 2 pints/1.1litre/5 cups of just-boiled water and let the tea cool. Clean wooden furniture or floors with a cloth soaked in the tea and squeezed out. Then dry it with an old towel.

- **Give white lace or clothes an 'antique' colour** – put 6 black-tea teabags into a large basin, add 2 pints/1.1litre/5 cups of just-boiled water and let the tea cool. Immerse the lace or clothing and soak for at least 10 minutes. The longer you leave it, the deeper the degree of the resulting ivory, ecru or beige colour.

- **Make a scented sachet for your wardrobe or bedroom drawers** – remove and dry the contents of used teabags, then use them to fill small cotton bags.

- **Shine mirrors** – make a strong brew of tea, let it cool, then use a cloth soaked in it, and squeezed out, to clean mirrors. Polish the mirror with a soft, lint-free cloth.

- **Tell fortunes** – some people claim they have a gift for using the pattern of tea leaves in the bottom of a cup to 'tell a person's fortune'. Such a fortune teller is probably either a charlatan or so sensitive to a person's feelings and, perhaps, knowledgeable about their circumstances and about life in general, that they can make a good attempt at predicting their future.

CHAPTER SEVEN

Recipes

The flavours of different teas and herb teas can add touches of magic to sweet and savoury dishes, as well as to drinks.

There are myriad ways of using teas. For example, you could use a tea to:

- Soak porridge oats overnight: try an Assam tea for malty, biscuity flavours or roasted corn tea for malty notes and slight sweetness.
- Add to a salad dressing: try adding ½ teaspoon per person of the powdered Japanese green tea called *matcha*.
- Add to the water when boiling or steaming vegetables: try roasted corn tea for pumpkin.
- Add to the water when boiling pasta: try black tea or roasted barley tea.
- Add to soup: try Darjeeling tea, dong quai or ginseng tea for chicken soup.
- Whizz with fruit to make a tea smoothie: try Assam tea with kiwis or linden-blossom tea with strawberries.
- Add to a vegetable or meat casserole: try green tea or rosemary or thyme tea.
- Make a savoury jelly: try Asssam tea jelly with beef; mint tea

jelly with lamb; and rosemary or thyme tea jelly with pork.

- Make a sweetened jelly to serve with cream or ice cream: try Darjeeling tea or hibiscus or peppermint tea.
- Soak dried fruits such as prunes or apricots: try black tea for prunes and roasted barley tea for apricots.
- Freeze into ice cubes for soft or alcoholic drinks: try green tea or an everyday herb tea such as chamomile or elderflower.
- Make ice lollies: try sweetened *Keemun* tea or roasted barley or hibiscus tea.
- Serve sweetened and cold, with ice cubes, as iced tea: try a Nilgiri tea since unlike certain other black teas it won't cloud as it cools; flavour it with lemon. Or try a hibiscus, lemon balm, lemongrass or peppermint tea.

Here are some recipes to try. Please note:

- Each recipe serves 4.
- 1 tsp (teaspoon) = 5ml; 1 tbsp (tablespoon) = 15ml; 1 cup = 240ml/8fl oz
- All fruit and vegetables are medium-sized unless otherwise stated.
- All eggs are medium (US large) unless otherwise stated.
- If using a fan oven, reduce the recommended temperature recommended by 20°C/68°F.

Main dishes

Tea and herb tea can be surprisingly good when added to certain recipes for fish, poultry and meat. Here are some examples.

PLAICE WITH LEMON BALM

The stronger the flavour of a fish, the more pronounced that of the tea or herb tea needed in the recipe. This one partners lemon balm with plaice, but green tea would be a good alternative. Another good combination is *Lapsang Souchong* with mackerel fillets. During cooking, the fish releases moisture that combines with the tea or herb tea to make a brew that imbues it with additional flavour.

675g/1½–2lb plaice fillets
2 tbsp dried or 4 tbsp fresh lemon balm
50g/2oz/½ stick butter
Salt and freshly ground black pepper
225g/8oz/1 cup cherry tomatoes

Preheat the oven to 180°C/350°F/gas 4.

Tear off a piece of aluminium foil large enough to wrap the fillets and put it onto a baking tray. Brush the foil with a little cooking oil.

Put the fillets onto the foil and cover each side of the fillets with lemon balm leaves. Dot each fillet with butter and sprinkle with salt and black pepper. Place the cherry tomatoes around the fillets.

Bake in the oven for 20 minutes.

ROSEMARY TEA AND CHICKEN CASSEROLE

Rosemary goes wonderfully with chicken. If you use it as a tea, there won't be any fiddly leaves in the creamy sauce of this casserole. If you prefer a lower-calorie version, use skinless chicken breasts and half-fat crème fraîche.

> 8 chicken breasts with skin
> 180ml/6fl oz/¾ cup extra virgin olive oil
> 2 onions, finely sliced
> 2 sticks celery, finely chopped
> 4 cloves garlic, finely chopped
> 720ml/24fl oz/3 cups hot rosemary tea
> 180ml/6fl oz/¾ cup crème fraîche

Preheat the oven to 180°C/350°F/gas 4.

Put the olive oil into a heavy-based casserole and heat it on the hob. Add the onions, celery and garlic and fry gently, stirring occasionally, until they begin to soften; do not brown. Add the chicken breasts and fry, turning occasionally, for a further 3 minutes.

Strain the hot rosemary tea into the casserole and bring to the boil. Cover the pot, put it into the oven and bake for 1¼ hours, turning the breasts after 30–40 minutes. Stir in the crème fraîche 10 minutes before the end of cooking. Serve hot with new potatoes and cabbage or other greens.

TEA-MARINATED STEAK

Marinating beef in black tea helps tenderise it, thanks to the tannins in tea. The smoky flavour of *Lapsang souchong* tea complements the flavour of beef very well.

4 steaks, each weighing 175–225g/6-8oz
600ml/20 fl oz/2½ cups strong *Lapsang souchong* tea

Put the steaks into a bowl, cover with the tea and leave to marinate for 1 hour.

Grill the steaks or fry them in a pan with a little extra virgin olive oil and butter until done to your liking.

Desserts and breads

Tea is well known as an ingredient of old favourite teatime treats such as brack, a traditional Irish spicy tea bread, and fruity tea loaf. But you can also use tea or herb tea in scones and cakes as well as in desserts such as jellies, sorbets, granitas and ice creams.

TEA LOAF

This quick and easy loaf is lovely with butter and jam – and a cup of tea!

    250g/8oz/1½ cups dried sultanas
    250g/8oz/1½ cups dried currants
    270ml/9fl oz/about 1 cup lukewarm strong black tea
    200g/7oz/1 cup soft light brown sugar
    225g/8oz/2cups self-raising flour
    1 tsp dried powdered cinnamon
    ½ tsp dried powdered nutmeg
    1 egg, beaten

Preheat the oven to 175ºC/325ºF/gas 3. Lightly butter a 10x22cm/5x9in loaf tin.

Put the sultanas, currants, tea and sugar into a large bowl, stir well, cover with a clean tea cloth and leave to soak overnight.

Stir in the self-raising flour, cinnamon and nutmeg, followed by the beaten egg.

Transfer the mixture to the loaf tin and bake for 1¼ hours or until a skewer inserted into the loaf comes out clean.

Serve sliced and spread with butter.

ROASTED BARLEY TEA SCONES

You could, of course, make scones from barley flour, but the roasted barley tea used here gives ordinary wheat flour a particularly delicious flavour. This recipe makes 8–10 scones. The secret to making good scones is to handle the dough as little as possible.

450g/1lb self-raising flour
2 heaped tsp baking powder
75g/3oz butter
50g/2oz caster sugar
2 large eggs, beaten
120ml/4fl oz/½ cup strong roasted barley tea
120ml/4fl oz/½ cup milk

Preheat the oven to 220°C/425°F/gas 7.

Lightly butter a baking tray.

Put the flour and baking powder into a large bowl. Add the butter and rub it in with your fingers until the mixture looks like fine bread-crumbs. Stir in the sugar.

Put the eggs into another bowl and beat them. Stir in the roasted barley tea and the milk. Reserve 2 tablespoons of the mixture. Gradually stir the rest into the flour, butter and sugar mixture to make a soft, moist and sticky dough.

On a lightly floured surface, with a rolling pin roll out the dough about ½–1in/1–2cm thick. Cut out the scones with a 2in/5cm cutter; avoid twisting the cutter so that the scones will rise more evenly.

Quickly and gently gather the remaining dough into a ball, roll it out and cut out more scones. Repeat as necessary.

Put the scones on the baking tray and brush with the reserved egg mixture.

Bake for 10–15 minutes until the scones are well risen and golden. Put them on a wire rack, cover with a clean tea towel (to help them stay moist) and let them cool completely.

Serve with butter and strawberry jam.

JAPANESE GREEN TEA ICE CREAM

This ice cream's beautiful green colour is completely natural as it comes from powdered Japanese green tea.

1 tbsp *matcha* green tea powder
3 tbsp hot water
180ml/6fl oz/¾ cup milk
2 egg yolks
100g/4oz/¾ cup caster sugar
180ml/6fl oz/¾ cup double cream, whipped

Put the *matcha* powder into a bowl and stir in the hot water.

Put the egg yolks into a pan and lightly beat them. Stir in the sugar. Gradually stir in the milk.

Gently heat the mixture, stirring constantly. When it has thickened, remove the pan from the heat and stand it in a container of cold water and ice cubes.

Stir in the green tea powder mixed with water, then the cream.

Either pour the mixture into an ice-cream maker and freeze it according to the ice-cream maker's instructions. Or pour the mixture into a container, cover it and put it into the freezer, stirring several times as it freezes.

Drinks

There's no need to stick with plain black tea with milk and, perhaps, sugar, when for the sake of a little experimentation you could be enjoying all manner of blended or flavoured teas. Here are just a few ideas.

MASALA CHAI

Very popular in India, this drink is made by boiling strong tea made from a dark, full-bodied type of tea such as an Assam with water, milk and several spices, perhaps including aniseed, cardamom, cinnamon, cloves, ginger and even chillies. You could use powdered dried ginger although fresh ginger is less pungent.

720ml/24fl oz/3 cups water

4 green cardamom pods (or 2 black cardamom if you prefer its smoky flavour)

1 cinnamon stick

4 tsp grated fresh ginger root

2 tsp dried black tea

240ml/8fl oz/1 cup milk

Freshly grated nutmeg

Put the water, cardamom, cinnamon and ginger into a pan and simmer, covered, for 10 minutes. Add the black tea and simmer, covered, for another 10 minutes. Add the milk and simmer for 1 minute more. Strain and sprinkle with nutmeg.

SEVEN-FLOWER TEA

Simple to make and delightful to drink! You can vary your selection of flowers and sweeten the tea if you like with honey or sugar.

Small pinch of each of 7 types of dried flower, chosen from
    calendula, chamomile, elderflower, hibiscus, jasmine, lavender,
    lime blossom, red clover and rosehip
420ml/14fl oz/1¾ cups boiling water

Put the dried flowers into a pan, add the boiling water, steep for 10 minutes, then reheat gently, if necessary, and strain.

RELAXING TEA

Try this wonderfully scented herb tea when you feel you need to put your feet up and have some time out.

1 pinch lavender
½ tsp lemon balm
½ tsp lime blossom
a few shreds of orange peel
1 pinch chamomile
480ml/16fl oz/2 cups boiling water

Put the lavender, lemon balm, lime blossom, orange peel and chamomile into a pan, add the boiling water, steep for 10 minutes, then reheat gently, if necessary, and strain.

TIM'S HOT PUNCH

This recipe is always welcome when groups of friends gather on a cold winter's day.

2 black-tea teabags
900ml/1½ pints/3½ cups boiling water
zest and juice of 1 lemon
2 cloves
1 cinnamon stick
600ml/1 pint/2½ cups red wine
2 tbsp clear honey
1 tbsp sugar

Put the teabags into a bowl, add the boiling water, lemon zest and juice, cloves and cinnamon stick, stir and steep for 20 minutes.

Line a sieve with kitchen paper and strain the liquid into a pan. Stir in the wine, honey and sugar and heat the punch without letting it come to the boil. Serve in warmed glasses.

Useful websites

Here are some of the organisations concerned with tea around the world.

AUSTRALIA
National Herbalists Association of Australia
www.nhaa.org.au
Offers a list of practitioners.

Austral Herbs
www.australherbs.com.au/
Sells teas and herbs.

FRANCE
Mariage frères
Branches in France, Germany and the UK.
www.mariagefreres.com
Sells teas, tea blends, tea-making accessories and tea-related gifts.

UNITED KINGDOM
G Baldwin & Co
www.baldwins.co.uk
Sells herbs.

Whole Foods Market
Also has stores in Canada and the US.
www.wholefoodsmarket.com
Sells teas.

The National Institute of Medical Herbalists
www.nimh.org.uk
Offers a list of practitioners.

Twinings
www.twinings.co.uk
Sells a wide range of teas and herb teas.

USA
American Bulk Herbs
www.bulkherbsusa.com
Sells herbs.

American Herbalists Guild
www.americanherbalistsguild.com
Offers a list of practitioners.

INDEX